THE UNABASHED
GARLIC &
ONION
Lover's
INTERNATIONAL
COOKBOOK

SUNNY BAKER
MICHELLE SBRAGA

Avery Publishing Group
Garden City Park, New York

Text Illustrator: John Wincek
Cover Designers: William Gonzalez, Rudy Shur and Phaedra Mastrocola
Front Cover Photo: Superstock, New York, NY
Typesetter: Elaine McCaw
In-House Editor: Marie Caratozzolo
Printer: Paragon Press, Honesdale, PA

Avery Publishing Group
120 Old Broadway
Garden City Park, NY 11020
1-800-548-5757

Library of Congress Cataloging-in-Publication Data

Baker, Sunny.
   The unabashed garlic & onion lover's international cookbook : a
robust collection of classic & contemporary garlic & onion recipes
from around the world / by Sunny Baker and Michelle Sbraga.
          p.   cm.
   Includes index.
   ISBN 0-89529-785-X
   1. Cookery (Garlic)   2. Cookery (Onions)   Cookery,
International.   4. Garlic.   5. Onions.   I. Sbraga, Michelle.
   II. Title.
TX819.G3B35   1997
641.6'525—dc21   97-6063
                                                             CIP

Contents

To the cast of thousands,
who shed their skins to be a part of this book.
And to our own families,
who made the "sacrifice" to be part of the story.

Preface

Fresh onions and garlic, which are available all year long in grocery stores and produce markets, are so abundant that most of us tend to take them for granted. Automatically we pick up a few onions and a bulb or two of garlic, but we don't pay much attention to them. They seem pretty ordinary . . . ho hum. But as prolific users of these products we know that it's not onions and garlic that are ordinary or ho hum, it's our meals without them.

Cooking with garlic and onions is an earthy pleasure. Whether peeling, smashing, mincing, or slicing, working with these flavorful bulbs gives us feelings of anticipation that no other ingredients can match. Few meals can be considered complete without their touch. They are favorite flavorings in nearly every type of cuisine. They add pungency to salsas and relishes, mellow richness to breads and steamed vegetables, and tantalizing spiciness to pastas and other entrées. And in such dishes as onion soup and baked garlic, these flavorful bulbs can stand on their own with ease. Along with their culinary prowess, garlic and onions are praised today, as they have been throughout history, for their medicinal qualities.

Because we are among those for whom life without garlic and onions would be unthinkable, we have written *The Unabashed Garlic & Onion Lover's International Cookbook*. This comprehensive volume is a compilation of our favorite international recipes that feature onions, garlic, and all of their relatives—including shallots, scallions, leeks, chives, and elephant garlic.

Through updated recipe classics and fresh innovations that have been developed specifically for this book, the humble onion and garlic are elevated to new taste sensations. From revealing the role of these savory plants in history, to sharing tips on growing them in any climate, to expounding their nutritional and medicinal value, and finally to using them in international cuisine, this book tells the whole story about these indispensable vegetables.

Introduction

Onions and garlic play a major role in today's healthful, natural cuisine. For only a few calories and no fat or cholesterol, these wonderful plants (alliums) impart flavor, vitamins, and other health benefits to meals. Onions and garlic add a subtle flavor of their own to foods, accentuating the taste and enjoyment of meals. Joined with other savory seasonings and fragrant herbs, they help us cut down on the use of salt and fats in our diets.

The inspiration for a book dedicated to onions and garlic comes from their year-round availability and universal appeal. Not too long ago, only white or yellow onions or onion powder and flakes were commonly available on supermarket shelves. Most of the garlic consumed was in powder or salt form, and "fresh" garlic came sealed in cellophane. These packaged forms are still available and used today, but in light of the switch to fresher, health-conscious foods, supermarkets and produce stands now carry mounds of fresh garlic and an impressive array of onion varieties. Sweet specialty onions such as Vidalias, Walla Wallas, and Mauis are becoming more and more commonplace on grocery shelves.

Onions and garlic are in greater demand in the kitchen than any other vegetable, but it is amazing how little people really know about these indispensable bundles of flavor. In addition to exploring the use of common onions and garlic in international cuisines, *The Unabashed Garlic & Onion Lover's International Cookbook* also intrigues gourmands with recipes that call for their close relatives, including shallots, chives, leeks, and elephant garlic.

The recipes presented in this book will appeal to a broad base of cooks ranging from the traditional to the adventurous. Both novice cooks and established gourmets will find recipes that appeal to their diverse culinary interests. All of the recipes are low in fat and sugar, and feature healthful, natural ingredients.

Whether the onion is sweet-tasting or biting hot, or the garlic is powerfully pungent or mellow-roasted, both are worldwide favorites. Standing on their own in featured roles, or adding a flavorful accent to crisp salads, savory entrées, or scrumptious sauces, onions and garlic are essentials in virtually every cuisine. So read on and enjoy! We promise you the trip will be worth it!

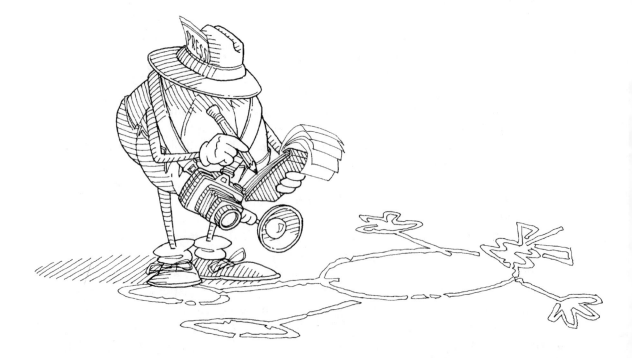

Chapter 1

The Spicy Story of Onions and Garlic

Yes, we cried over writing this book. But the tears were those of joy—the joy of cooking with garlic and onions. There is hardly a meal we make that doesn't have a foundation of leeks, a litany of chopped sweet onion, or, at the very least, a sprinkling of chives.

Many international cuisines are onion or garlic based. Battuto, for example, a simple mixture of chopped onion with a bit of parsley, olive oil, and garlic, is the foundation for many Italian pasta sauces, soups, and risottos. Some diced carrots, celery, or anything else that pleases the chef's fancy also can be added. Soffritto is battuto that has been carefully sautéed until the onions become translucent and the garlic takes on a little color.

The French employ onions or garlic in virtually everything—from sauces and stocks to bouillon and aspics. They are the basis of French cooking. The same can be said of the cuisines of Germany, Hungary, India, Britain, Scotland, and Australia.

Although common yellow or white onions are seldom used in Chinese cooking, scallions and garlic are quite popular. Paired with ginger for that distinctive Far Eastern flavor, scallions and garlic are common ingredients in stir-fry dishes. Almost anywhere in the world, you'll find onions or garlic or both playing a central role.

THE STORY OF THE ONION FAMILY—READ IT AND WEEP!

Onions belong to the genus *Allium* of the family *Liliaceae* (related to lilies). Common cultivated onions are varieties of the species *Allium cepa*. This species, probably native to southwestern Asia, has been cultivated in temperate and sub-

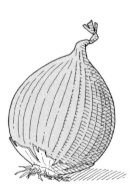

Yellow Onion

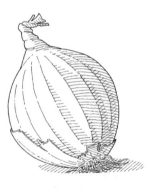

White Onion

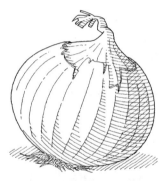

Spanish Onion

tropical regions for thousands of years. In China, it is documented that onions were cultivated more than 5,000 years ago. In the Middle East, the onion has existed for over 4,000 years. And onions are mentioned in the earliest writings of the Indian Vedics.

Common onions, which no longer exist in the wild, were cultivated by the ancient Egyptians. The Romans spread the use of onions and garlic to much of Northern Europe. From Europe, the onion was brought by the Spanish colonists to the New World.

The true onion is a bulb-bearing plant. It has long, hollow leaves and a thick base that makes up most of the bulb. Its white or pink flowers, which are born in umbels, have six sepals, six petals, six stamens, and a solitary pistil. In the varieties known as top onions, the flowers are supplanted by bulblets, which may be grown to obtain new plants.

All relatives of the onion have a similar, distinctive aroma. This "bouquet" (and their great taste) comes from sulfurous, volatile oils. It is these sulfurous compounds that dissolve in water to produce sulfuric acid, which is produced when onion fumes or oils come into contact with the eyes. This is why a cut onion brings tears to one's eyes.

THE ONION FAMILY CAST OF CHARACTERS

Many relatives of the common *Allium cepa* are worth experimenting with in the kitchen, including the nodding wild onion (*Allium cernuum*); the shallot (*Allium ascalonicum*); the chive (*Allium schoenoprasum*); and the common leek (*Allium ampeloprasum*). The total onion genus contains about 700 species, usually with underground bulbs and long, slender leaves that start at the ground (basal leaves). We describe only the commonly used alliums here; but you may meet their other tasty relatives in your travels around the world or across the street in your favorite grocery store or gourmet shop.

Yellow Onions

The most common onions used in cooking are the yellow storage onions. Ranging in size from very small to medium-large, these onions, when cut, usually bring tears to one's eyes. Cooking, however, transforms this onion's hot, biting flavor into mellow sweetness. A dry onion with a brown, thick papery skin, the yellow onion is a real workhorse. Use it when subtlety is not a priority.

White Onions

Although they can be used interchangeably with their yellow cousins, white onions are sharper and cleaner-flavored. Their shelf life, however, is slightly shorter than the yellow onion because proportionally they have more water and they lack the pigment that protects them from mold. Initially, a white onion may taste sweet, but within moments, the sulfur kicks in and the heat appears.

Spanish Onions

The large, yellow Spanish onions are slightly higher in water content than ordinary yellow and white storage onions; they are also sweeter, crisper, and more perishable. Spanish onions, which have taken the place of the Bermuda line that died out in the 1980s, have just enough heat to remind you of their Latin heritage. They are common substitutes for the more expensive, less available sweet specialty onions, such as the Vidalia, Walla Walla, and Maui.

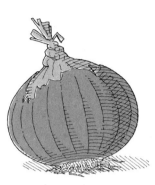

Red Onion

Red Onions

Similar in character to Spanish onions, red onions are sharp, sweet, and pungent. Their papery outer skin is very thick, and their texture is coarser than other onions. Slices of raw red onion add a colorful statement to any salad or antipasto, as well as a wide variety of main dishes. Once cooked, however, these onions lose their vibrant red hue.

Boiling Onions

Small white or yellow onions are often referred to as boiling onions. Generally about 2 inches in diameter, boiling onions are best left whole and boiled or simmered.

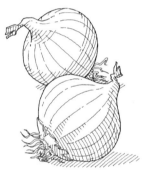

Boiling Onions

Pearl Onions

Tiny pearl onions are typically 1 to $1^{1}/_{4}$ inches in diameter, with outer skins that are thin and transparent. They are crisp and surprisingly sweet. Pearl onions are great when pickled, marinated, or skewered on a kebab. Small boiling onions can be substituted for pearl in most recipes.

Sweet Specialty Onions

Sweet onions have a very high water content, which makes them mild-tasting and sweet. They are extremely crisp and fairly perishable. Sold under a variety of regional monikers, Vidalia, Maui, Texas, Arizona, and Walla Walla are the best-known. These sweet onions are available seasonally, as their growing season is shorter than it is for common storage onions. Most varieties are yellow in color and resemble slightly flattened globes. The larger the onion the sweeter its taste. Most are deliciously flavorful when raw and delicately sweet when cooked. Because they caramelize nicely, sweet onions are ideal in sauces, sautés, and soups.

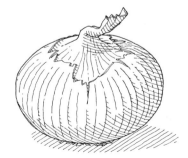

Vidalia Onion

THOSE GARLIC RELATIVES

Prized for at least 5,000 years, garlic likely originated in the steppes of Central Asia. Inscriptions on the pyramids at Giza told of the large amounts of garlic that had been consumed by the workers who built them. And, in order to build and maintain their strength, ancient Olympic athletes were said to eat garlic in large quantities.

Like the related onion, garlic has small, six-part, whitish flowers borne on umbels. The garlic fruit is a capsule containing black, kidney-shaped seeds. The bulb, which has a strong characteristic odor and taste, is covered with a papery skin and may be broken into constituent bulblets, called cloves. The tender young shoots of the garlic plant are called "green garlic" and can be used for a milder garlic flavor in many recipes.

Although the common cloved garlic and the colossal elephant garlic are the types most often used to season foods, other less-common varieties—British wild garlic, American wild garlic, and field garlic of both Europe and the Americas—are also used as seasonings. North American false garlic, or crow poison, is closely related to garlic but lacks the characteristic garlic odor.

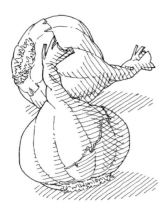

Cloved Garlic

Cloved Garlic

Common cloved garlic, classified as *Allium sativum*, includes many varieties. Their papery bulbs span the color spectrum from white and creamy yellow to red and purple. California varieties are the most common, but the Mexican or Italian purple, and the south Australian white are also generally available. Large-cloved varieties include the giant Russian, purple New Zealand, and the Glenlarge, which can be grown almost anywhere and at any time of the year.

When buying garlic, look for bulbs that are plump and firm with no brown spots. Whole garlic has no smell. It isn't until the cloves are cut or crushed that their characteristic smell is released. Whole cloves that are cooked result in honeyed morsels that are mellow and nutty in taste. Cut garlic is always more pungent, even after it is cooked. Slow-roasting or sautéing garlic brings out its best cooked flavor. Just be careful not to burn the cloves. Burnt garlic is acrid and bitter.

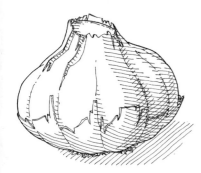

Elephant Garlic

Elephant Garlic

Although its cloves are several times larger than common cloved garlic, elephant garlic is milder and more subtle flavored. Its taste is more like a leek than garlic, and because of this mildness, some cooks refuse to substitute it for the stronger-flavored cloved varieties. Others appreciate its gentle flavor. You can find bulbs of elephant garlic in many grocery stores and most gourmet or specialty food shops.

OTHER MEMBERS OF THE ALLIUM FAMILY

The allium family's kissing cousins—scallions, leeks, chives, and shallots—offer their distinctive characteristics to a wide variety of dishes.

Scallions

Also called green onions, flavorful scallions are young bulb onions that are harvested before their bulbs have developed an outer skin. They are sold with their green leaves attached and are usually about 10 inches long. Sweet and mild-tasting, scallions are delicious both raw and cooked, and their white stems as well as their leaves are edible. If scallions are allowed more time in the ground, their bulbs become a bit larger and they are known are creaming onions.

Sold by the bunch, scallions are affordably priced and available year round, so we use them liberally. In the cuisines of China and Japan, they are a mainstay. Scallions are the only onion family members that should be stored in the refrigerator, where they will keep for a week.

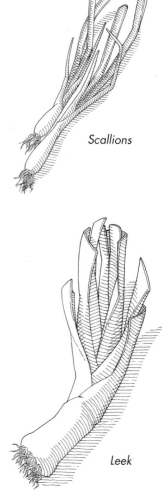

Scallions

Leeks

Resembling a large, fat scallion, the versatile leek is actually a member of the lily family, but in flavor, it is more like a mild cousin of the onion. Cultivated for thousands of years, leeks are easy to grow but require a long growing season. Commonly used to flavor meats, soups, and stews, leeks are easy to digest and a popular ingredient in international cuisines. We like to add chopped tender leeks to salads (in place of onions or scallions) and top with a simple vinaigrette.

Use the leek's tender white bulb only, making sure to discard its tough green stalks. And be aware that leeks are characteristically filled with grit and sand; they must be thoroughly cleaned before they are prepared.

Leek

Shallots

These tender, delicate members of the onion family have clustered bulbs that are wrapped in bronze skin. They grow easily in a fashion similar to garlic, and should be stored in a cool, dry place. Increasingly popular, shallots are now commonly available in most grocery stores. Possessing just a hint of garlic flavor, shallots are onions without the harsh taste (we characterize them as half garlic and half onion).

Shallots make a superb base for sauces and they are a splendid addition to omelets. They vary in flavor according to variety. Often sweet and delicate, fresh raw shallots also can be strong-flavored and quite hot. When slow-roasted, shallots caramelize nicely. Fresh shallots are best added to dishes that are mild-flavored. Their sweet delicacy should be showcased, not buried in overpowering flavors.

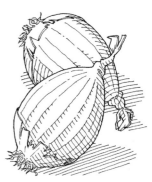

Shallots

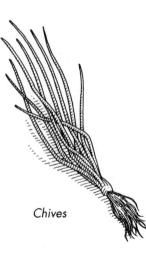

Chives

Chives

Mild-tasting and delicate, chives are grassy flavored with just a hint of onion and no heat. Their slender hollow leaves and flowers are edible and are commonly used to garnish soups, salads, and egg dishes. As cooking greatly diminishes the flavor of chives, they are best added to cold dishes or sprinkled on a dish just before serving. Although chives are sweeter and more tender than scallions, minced scallions are often substituted for chives as a garnish.

The garlic chive, with its distinctive garlic flavor, is heartier than the regular chive. Not readily available in most grocery stores, garlic chives are easily grown in home herb gardens. Because of their hearty natures, garlic chives can be used in place of garlic or scallions in recipes that don't require lengthy cooking times.

ONIONS AND GARLIC ARE HEALTH FOODS

Do you know what you get when you take a bite out of an onion? You get a variety of vitamins and minerals—including a substantial jolt of vitamin C and dietary fiber—with only a few calories, no fat, no cholesterol, and almost no salt. Not only do onions and garlic enhance the taste of foods, nutritionally, they are foods worth eating. Take a look at the table below for the nutritional analysis of a medium-sized yellow onion.

Throughout history, cultures that have incorporated onions in their cuisine also have recognized their healing powers. Onions were a common folk remedy in the 1800s for various illnesses—the stronger the onion, the more likely it was to cure what ailed you.

Nutritional Analysis of a 5-Ounce Yellow Onion

Calories	60
Protein	1.2 gms
Carbohydrates	14.0 gms
Fat	0.0 gms
Cholesterol	0.0 gms
Sodium	10.0 mg
Potassium	200.0 mg
Vitamin C	11.9 mg
Vitamin B_6	120.1 mcg
Calcium	38.0 mg
Phosphorus	40.3 mg
Dietary Fiber	2.8 gms

In Ancient Egypt, onion juice was prescribed for coughs, colds, and stomach ailments. It was rubbed on cuts, acne, animal bites, powder burns, and warts. It even was used to treat ear infections.

While onions may not grow hair or cure blindness as the Romans claimed, mounting scientific evidence suggests that the therapeutic powers of the allium family are real. A number of chemicals—allicin, in particular—found naturally in onions, have been scientifically proven to aid in both the prevention and the treatment of various blood disorders. When included as a regular part of the diet, studies have shown that onions, shallots, leeks, chives, and garlic can help minimize circulatory problems by reducing cholesterol levels in the blood.

Although your friends might find chewing onions offensive, the technique might prevent a sore throat during cold season. Studies have confirmed the bacteria-killing, antiseptic properties of onions, and it is believed that chewing raw onions for five minutes will sterilize the mouth and throat. Onions also have the ability to loosen phlegm, and they are a natural diuretic.

The National Cancer Institute has included all of the onion family members onto its list of cruciferous vegetables, calling them "promising agents in combating certain types of cancer, in particular, stomach cancer." Curecetin, an antioxidant recognized as a cancer-blocking agent by the National Institutes of Health, is present in the entire allium family. Recently, garlic was named by the National Cancer Institute as one of the best natural cancer preventives. Researchers have also noted that onions may prevent blood clots and reduce blood pressure. Certain onion compounds act like the chemical anticlotting agents that are frequently used to stabilize heart-attack patients.

The inclusion of onions and garlic in your diet may help combat some serious health problems, but even if they didn't, they still taste good.

GROWING ONIONS

We always prefer fresh onions and garlic over dried or jarred varieties. And what better way to assure that the vegetables you eat are free from pesticides and other chemicals than to grow your own?

Onions are easy to grow in almost any climate. In a home garden or greenhouse, onions and scallions are most commonly grown from sets. Sets are small, dried bulblets that have been raised from seeds the previous year and picked while young. Each immature bulblet in the set produces a mature onion during the growing season. Although seeds are also available, we prefer to use sets because they are easy to plant and rarely fail to produce. Sets for many onion varieties are available in large gardening departments and nurseries.

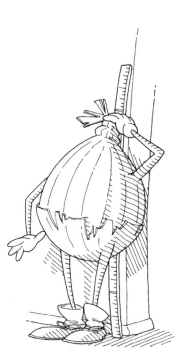

Onions are adaptable to different temperatures and can be planted year-round as long as the soil is rich and moist and the ground is not frozen. Onions raised commercially in warm areas are planted as winter crops and are milder in taste and odor than onions planted during the summer in cooler regions. In most home gardens, onion varieties are best planted four to six weeks before the last frost in the spring or late summer for a fall crop.

Sets are planted in a furrow or hole about 2 inches deep. If the sets are to be grown to mature onions, the space between each set should be about 4 inches. Onions require rich soil and an open, sunny area. Add a natural fertilizer (such as compost or manure) on a monthly basis for the best-tasting, healthiest onions. The soil should be kept loose and free from weeds, and it should be well-drained. Onions also need plenty of water, especially when they are young.

About four months after planting, your onions should be ready to harvest. Onions should be allowed to ripen in the ground until their tops begin to bend and break. You'll know when the bulbs are ready for harvest when the plant's leaves turn yellow and become limp. Carefully pull the onions from the ground and cut off their dead tops to within an inch of the bulb. Spread the onions out or hang them up to dry in an open area. Once their stems are somewhat shriveled, store the onions in open-mesh bags to prevent sprouting.

It is very important to keep your onions dry. Neck rot, caused by fungi, is one of the most serious infections of stored onions. Neck rot generally develops because onions have not been properly dried before storage or because the storage environment is too warm and moist. To avoid spoilage from fungi, store your onions in a cool, dry place with adequate ventilation. Onions stored in the refrigerator are likely to get damp and are subject to mold and fungi contamination.

GROWING GARLIC

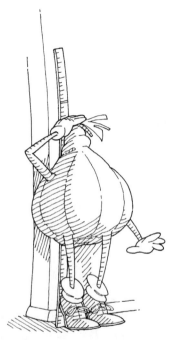

Garlic is fairly easy to grow. It thrives almost anywhere and under most conditions. Garlic likes cool winters and hot summers. Growing pungent garlic requires lots of sunlight and rich, well-drained soil. If your garden soil holds water, you may choose to construct a raised bed for your garlic.

Garlic cloves are used to grow garlic. (Some people refer to a garlic clove as a "tooth.") Choosing healthy bulbs will reduce the chances of fungal disease—the biggest problem when cultivating garlic. The bigger the clove, the better the start, and the more garlic you'll reap for your efforts. The cloves you plant should be firm, plump, and free from spots or mildew. You can buy garlic cloves almost anywhere.

Leaving on their papery skins, plant garlic cloves about 1 to 2 inches deep and about 4 inches apart with the pointed ends facing upward. A slightly alkaline soil is best. For the best results, the garlic cloves should be in chilled soil (below 50°F) early in their growing period. If the bulbs aren't chilled during this period, the cloves will be small and uneven, and they will have thin, papery skin.

In temperate areas, where winter temperatures fall below 50°F, but the ground does not freeze, garlic is best planted in the fall. In areas where the ground freezes solid, plant garlic in the spring, as the cloves may rot in frozen soil. In hot areas, chill the cloves for a month in the refrigerator before planting. If you live in a very hot climate, plant the cloves in midwinter when the ground is cool and not likely to warm up again until spring.

In order to produce large bulbs, garlic plants must be well-fed. Spread natural fertilizer over the soil when you plant your cloves, then feed them again when the young leaves begin to show through the topsoil.

Your first sight of the growing garlic will be dull green leaf tips that soon develop into long, flat leaves. Within a few months, a round, thick stalk will emerge and grow anywhere from $1^1/2$ to 3 feet in length. The stalk produces flowers that blossom in spectacular blues, purples, pinks, or whites. The flowers are edible and delicious in salads. In very cool climates, garlic plants may not flower, but they will still mature.

Among the garlic flowers you'll find tiny bulbs called bulbiles or bulblets. These should be removed to encourage bulb growth. Bulblets are very tasty and can be used in the same way as mature garlic cloves.

Garlic takes from five to nine months to mature, depending on the climate. When the stalks begin to wither and become yellow and leathery, the garlic is ready to harvest. Don't wait until the stalks wither completely, as you do with onion plants. And don't pull the bulbs out by their stalks, rather dig them from the ground.

Dry the harvested garlic in a well-ventilated area that is out of direct sunlight. It takes a few weeks to fully dry a crop. At all costs, avoid dampness. Moisture leads to mold and rot.

When the garlic is quite papery, you can braid the stalks and/or knot the plants together, or simply let the stalks hang in bunches. Alternatively, you can leave the bulbs on racks or store them in airy baskets. Never put them in the refrigerator. Properly stored, garlic will delight your tastebuds for months.

Don't use all of your garlic cloves in our recipes. Instead, save some individual cloves for next year's growing season. Keep the cloves dry and cool until planting time.

COOKING WITH ALLIUMS

Although jars of minced or chopped garlic and onions are readily available in most grocery stores, we avoid them. It's so easy to chop and peel these items, and they are so sturdy, we can't justify the flavor lost for the few seconds of saved preparation time. Our belief is that there is nothing like fresh.

When Cooking Onions

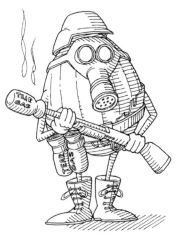

Of course, we cannot deny that cutting a fresh onion has its downside—bringing tears to one's eyes being the most obvious. The good news is that we can help you combat those tears. In order to keep from crying when cutting those onions, try one of the following tricks:

• Chill the onions for at least 30 minutes before cutting them.
• Cut the onion under cold running water.
• Place a recently blown-out match in your mouth while cutting the onion.
• Turn on a fan or exhaust vent to reduce the lingering fumes.
• Drop a peeled onion into boiling water for a minute before cutting it.

For the best, freshest flavor, cut onions as close to cooking time or serving time as possible. When cooking onions, whether sautéing them on the stovetop or slow-roasting them in the oven, use low or medium heat. Intense heat may cause the onions to taste bitter. On the other hand, when searing onions, use high heat for a short amount of time to produce the best flavor. And to keep onions crunchy when serving them raw, marinate them in a mild vinegar for 30 minutes.

To alleviate the lingering odor of onions on your work surface, rub the surface with salt and lemon or white vinegar before washing it with hot water and soap.

When Cooking Garlic

Garlic has two quite distinct flavors. It is strong and pungent when raw, and mellow and nutty when cooked. Cooked garlic is sweetest when it is slow-roasted or sautéed lightly.

When sautéing garlic, be sure to do so slowly and just enough to soften it. Once garlic begins to brown, watch out. Within the blink of an eye, it can burn. And burnt garlic is bitter-tasting. Slow-roasting garlic is another cooking method that brings out its flavorful sweetness. When slow-roasted, the pungent cloves are transformed into caramelized sweetened morsels that add flavor to a number of dishes. The roasted cloves also can be spread on crusty bread instead of butter. See the recipe on page 25.

The best way to crush garlic is with a garlic crusher. The cloves are placed in the chamber—papery skin and all—and crushed. For the most flavor, always choose to crush garlic rather than chop it.

And, as with onions, clean your work surface with a little salt and lemon juice or white vinegar before washing it with hot soapy water. This will alleviate any garlic smell.

WHEN PREPARING THE RECIPES IN THIS BOOK

The international recipes presented in this book support a healthy diet; most include little sugar and a minimum of fat. While spotlighting members of the allium family, we also feature a variety of healthful ingredients including tofu, beans, nuts, grains, fresh vegetables, chicken, and fish. There are no red meat dishes, and most of the recipes will suit vegetarians.

We recommend using fresh, organically grown produce whenever possible. And, when available, use fresh herbs, which impart full-flavor without the harshness that often characterizes the dried and bottled varieties. In the few recipes in which chicken stock is called for, feel free to substitute a vegetable stock if you prefer a strictly vegetarian cuisine.

When Measuring Garlic

Unless otherwise specified, when garlic is called for in this book's recipes, use medium-sized cloves. When a specific measurement is needed, use the following equivalents as your guide:

1 teaspoon	=	1 finely chopped medium clove
1 tablespoon	=	3 finely chopped medium cloves
$1/4$ cup	=	12 finely chopped medium cloves

When Measuring Onions

Cooking with onions does not require the precision necessary for measuring other ingredients, such as flour and spices. It is just fine to add a little more or a little less onion than our recipes call for. Just keep in mind that the cooking time may need adjusting.

When we call for a specific number of onions, we are referring to those that are medium-sized. If you prefer more onion flavor, feel free to use larger onions or increase the number of onions called for. When considering how many onions you'll need for a specific measurement, use the table on the following page as a guide.

Feel Free to Substitute

Don't feel limited by the specific type of onion or garlic called for in

Onion Equivalent Amounts

Size	Weight	Equivalent
Small	= 2 ounces	= $2/3$ cup coarsely chopped = $1/2$ cup sliced = $1/3$ cup grated = $1/4$ cup cooked
Medium	= 4 ounces	= 1 cup coarsely chopped = $3/4$ cup sliced = $2/3$ cup grated = $1/2$ cup cooked
Large	= 8 ounces	= 2 cups coarsely chopped = $1^{1}/2$ cups sliced = $1^{1}/3$ cups grated = 1 cup cooked
Very large	= 1 pound	= 4 cups coarsely chopped = 3 cups sliced = $2^{2}/3$ cups grated = 2 cups cooked

our recipes. Most allium family members can be substituted for each other. When a dish calls for scallions, try substituting chives, baby leeks, green garlic, or young shallot shoots. For recipes in which onions are sautéed, use milder-flavored shallots or leeks. Substitute red onions for yellow, and leeks for mild white onions.

"Take a Chance"

Every one of our recipes includes a "Take a Chance" section. This section offers helpful hints and guidelines to help you in your own creative manipulations of the recipes. We suggest that you jot down any recipe changes you make when creating a masterpiece. This will help you to remember it for the next time. And there will be a next time, we promise.

TIME TO GET STARTED

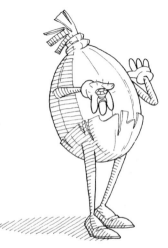

Remember, onions and garlic in any amount and combination can turn ordinary meals into culinary events that will bring tears of joy to your eyes. Now, let the tears flow . . . start chopping those onions and mincing that garlic. The world is at your fingertips.

Chapter 2

Appetizers
Jump-Start Your Meals

Garlic and onions can add zing to many appetizing treats from around the world. Their piquant taste leaves the diner asking for more. But be aware: when having guests for dinner, don't let them go overboard with the appetizers found in this chapter. You will run the risk of ruining their appetites for the other sensational onion and garlic creations that follow.

Red Onion Spread United States

We love this piquant jam on crackers or toasted bread as an appetizer. You can also spread it over chicken before cooking, or use it as a condiment.

8 cups chopped red onions

3 tablespoons soy margarine

3 tablespoons honey

2/3 cup concentrated fruit sweetener

1/2 cup cider vinegar

1/4 cup dry sherry

YIELD: 3 1/2 CUPS   PREPARATION TIME: 1 HOUR

1. Place the onions and margarine in a large saucepan over medium heat, and sauté for 5 minutes. Reduce the heat to low and add the remaining ingredients. Simmer the mixture, uncovered, for 30 to 45 minutes, or until it has thickened.

2. Pour the mixture into a sterilized heat-proof jar and seal. When cool, store in the refrigerator.

3. Serve the jam at room temperature.

TAKE A CHANCE:

• Use yellow onions instead of red.

• Add a dash of chili powder to the mixture.

Sour Cream Party Dip United States

Americans love their dip on chips, pretzels, and crisp vegetables. This one, made lively with chopped onion and bit of hot sauce, tastes great on everything.

2 cups nonfat sour cream

3/4 cup grated lowfat cheddar cheese

3 tablespoons finely chopped yellow or white onion

1/4 teaspoon hot sauce

YIELD: 2 3/4 CUPS   PREPARATION TIME: 1 HOUR

1. Mix all the ingredients together in a medium bowl. Cover and refrigerate for 1 hour.

2. Mix well and serve immediately.

TAKE A CHANCE:

• Replace the sour cream with equal parts yogurt and nonfat sour cream.

• Use 2 finely chopped scallions instead of the onion.

• Add 1/2 teaspoon finely chopped jalapeño or serrano chili pepper.

• Sprinkle with paprika or cayenne pepper before serving.

Spinach Dip Persia (Iran)

YIELD: 2 CUPS   PREPARATION TIME: 20 MINUTES

1. Place the oil in a skillet over medium heat. Add the onion and garlic and sauté for 1 minute. Add the cumin, curry powder, turmeric, and cinnamon, and sauté another minute. Add the spinach and cook 2 minutes, or until the spinach is wilted.

2. Remove the skillet from the heat, add the yogurt, and mix the ingredients together.

3. Serve immediately with chunks of bread, crackers, or fresh vegetables.

TAKE A CHANCE:

• Serve the dip in a hollowed-out loaf of round sourdough bread. Cut the bread into bite-sized pieces. Toast the pieces and use for dipping.

• Water chestnuts didn't grow anywhere near ancient Persia, but you can add a little crunch to this dip by adding $1/4$ cup of coarsely chopped ones.

*O*nions have long been a favorite ingredient in Middle Eastern cooking. In this recipe, the chunks of onion and garlic, along with fragrant spices, perfectly complement the tart taste of the spinach and yogurt.

1 tablespoon canola oil

1 small yellow or white onion, coarsely chopped

3 cloves garlic, coarsely chopped

1 teaspoon cumin

$1/2$ teaspoon curry powder

$1/2$ teaspoon turmeric

$1/8$ teaspoon cinnamon

$3 1/2$ cups fresh spinach, washed and coarsely chopped

1 cup plain yogurt

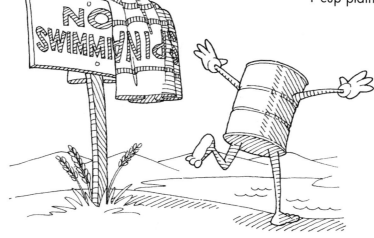

Baba Ghanoush Middle East

*W*e translate the Arabic name of this dish as *"roasted eggplant with plenty of garlic!" This favorite Middle Eastern treat is simply wonderful. Make plenty because it will go fast.*

1 large eggplant

5 cloves garlic, finely chopped

1/4 cup fresh lemon juice

1/2 cup tahini

1/2 teaspoon cumin

YIELD: 3 CUPS   PREPARATION TIME: 2 1/2 HOURS

1. Place the eggplant on a baking sheet, and pierce it several times with a fork. Bake the eggplant in a 350°F oven for 1 hour, or until it is soft. Turn the eggplant several times during baking.

2. When the eggplant is cool enough to handle, scoop out the insides and place it in a large bowl. Add the garlic, lemon juice, tahini, and cumin, and mix well. Cover and chill for 1 hour.

3. Mix well and serve immediately as a dip for fresh vegetables, a filling for pita bread, or a spread for crusty rolls.

TAKE A CHANCE:

- For a smoky flavor, roast the eggplant on a barbecue or over an open flame.

- Add one or more of the following to the mixture: 1 tablespoon minced onion, 1 minced jalapeño pepper, 1 teaspoon freshly grated lemon peel.

Guacamole Cups Mexico

YIELD: 8 SERVINGS   PREPARATION TIME: 1½ HOURS

1. Using a sharp knife, carefully cut the avocados in half and remove the pit.

2. With a spoon, gently scoop out the pulp and place it in a medium bowl. (Leave just enough avocado in the skins to help them retain their shape.) Rub the lime juice over the shells to keep them from turning black and set aside.

3. Mash the avocado with a fork or a large spoon until almost smooth. Add the onion and garlic and mix well.

4. Mound the guacamole into the shells. Garnish with tomatoes and cilantro and serve immediately.

TAKE A CHANCE:

• Use chopped shallots instead of onions.

• Add 2 to 3 seeded, finely chopped jalapeño peppers or a few drops of hot sauce.

• Use parsley instead of cilantro.

Served in their own shells, this guacamole is a treat on everything from warm tortilla chips to hamburgers. Traditional Mexican guacamole doesn't have garlic, but we can't seem to leave it out.

4 ripe avocados

1 teaspoon lime juice

½ cup finely minced onion

2 cloves garlic, crushed

2 tablespoons finely chopped fresh cilantro

2 tablespoons seeded and finely chopped tomatoes

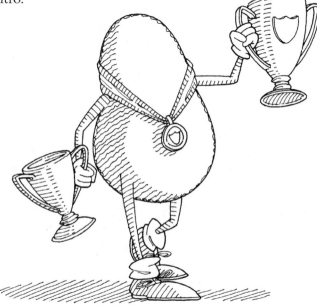

Garlic Yogurt Dip **United States**

Filled with fresh garlic and scallions, this yogurt-based dip is low in fat and calories. And it tastes good, too!

2/3 cup plain lowfat yogurt

3 cloves garlic, crushed

2 scallions, finely chopped

1/4 cup finely chopped fresh mint

3 tablespoons fresh lemon juice

1/4 teaspoon freshly ground black pepper

1/8 teaspoon paprika

YIELD: 1 CUP   PREPARATION TIME: 20 MINUTES

1. Mix all the ingredients, except the paprika, together in a bowl. Cover and set aside for 15 minutes. Do not refrigerate.

2. Garnish with paprika and serve with crackers or fresh vegetables. This flavorful dip is also good tucked into your favorite pita sandwich or spread on a Vegetable Hoagie (page 40).

TAKE A CHANCE:

• Add 3 tablespoons seeded and finely chopped cucumbers.

• Use equal parts lowfat yogurt and nonfat sour cream instead of all yogurt.

• Add 2 more teaspoons of lemon juice and use as a salad dressing over garden fresh tomatoes or cucumbers.

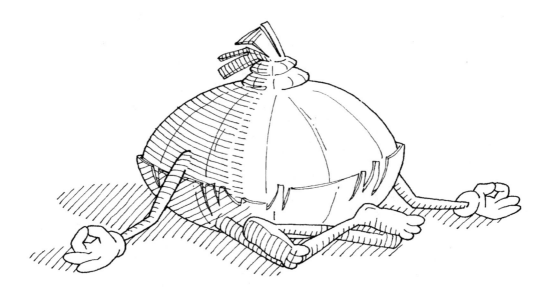

Bagna Cauda France

YIELD: 1 CUP   PREPARATION TIME: 20 MINUTES

1. Melt the margarine in a small saucepan over low heat. Add the olive oil and heat for 1 minute. Add the garlic and cook another minute.

2. Remove the pan from the heat, add the anchovies, and mix thoroughly. Return the pan to the heat and continue stirring until the anchovies dissolve.

3. Serve immediately with crusty French bread or raw vegetables.

TAKE A CHANCE:

• Add 1/4 teaspoon crushed red pepper.

Literally translated, bagna cauda means "hot bath." This wonderful dip from Provence is filled with garlic and not for the faint of heart.

1/2 cup soy margarine

1/4 cup extra-virgin olive oil

5 cloves garlic, crushed

5 anchovy fillets, coarsely chopped

Anchovy Spread France

YIELD: 3/4 CUP   PREPARATION TIME: 20 MINUTES

1. Place the shallots and garlic in a food processor and pulse until finely chopped. Add the vinegar and pulse 2 times. Add the anchovies and pulse until smooth.

2. With the motor running, add the oil in a slow stream. Add the parsley and blend 5 seconds.

3. Serve immediately on toasted bread or as dip for fresh vegetables.

TAKE A CHANCE:

• Use fresh lemon juice instead of vinegar.

• Use 2 scallions instead of the shallots.

Like its counterpart Bagna Cauda (above), this spread is redolent with the flavor of garlic and anchovies. Added are the fresh taste of shallots and the tang of red wine vinegar.

2 shallots, cut in half

4 cloves garlic

1 tablespoon red wine vinegar

8 anchovy fillets, chopped

3 tablespoons extra-virgin olive oil

3 sprigs parsley, finely chopped

Salsa Cruda Mexico

Living close to the Arizona-Mexico border, we serve salsa with everything.

5 large ripe tomatoes, seeded and coarsely chopped

$1/4$ cup finely chopped yellow or white onion

2 cloves garlic, finely chopped

2 large jalapeño peppers, seeded and finely chopped

$1/4$ cup finely minced cilantro

Juice of 2 fresh limes

YIELD: 1$1/2$ CUPS   PREPARATION TIME: 45 MINUTES

1. Place all of the ingredients in a glass bowl or jar and stir well. Cover and refrigerate at least 30 minutes.

2. Stir well before serving.

TAKE A CHANCE:

• Use 3 teaspoons fresh lemon juice instead of lime juice.

• Use serrano chili peppers instead of jalapeño peppers.

• Use $1/4$ cup minced green bell peppers instead of jalapeño peppers.

• Serve as a sauce over meat or egg dishes.

• Use over Baked Potatoes with Garlic Chives (page 131).

New World Popcorn United States

Americans are munching more and more popcorn each day. Garlic, scallions, and a variety of spices brought to the New World by the Conquistadors add piquant flavor to this favorite snack.

4 quarts fresh-popped popcorn

3 tablespoons soy margarine

3 cloves garlic, crushed

$1/2$ cup finely chopped scallions

$1/4$ teaspoon cayenne pepper

$1/4$ teaspoon paprika

YIELD: 4 QUARTS   PREPARATION TIME: 5 MINUTES

1. Melt the margarine in a small saucepan over low heat. Add the garlic and sauté for 1 minute. Add the cayenne pepper, paprika, and scallions, and sauté another minute.

2. Place the popcorn in a large bowl, drizzle with the melted margarine mixture, and mix well.

3. Serve immediately.

TAKE A CHANCE:

• Use chives instead of scallions.

• For an Italian taste, omit scallions, cayenne pepper, and paprika. Add $1/2$ tsp. dried oregano, $1/4$ tsp. dried thyme leaves, and $1/2$ cup finely chopped fresh parsley to the margarine. Toss with the popcorn and sprinkle with $1/4$ cup freshly grated Parmesan cheese.

Spiced Olives Morocco

YIELD: 2 CUPS   PREPARATION TIME: 3 HOURS

1. Mix all of the ingredients, except the olives, together in a large glass jar. Add the olives and mix well. If necessary, add more lemon juice or olive oil to completely cover the olives. Tightly close the jar and let stand for 3 hours or more.

2. Before serving, shake the jar well. Spoon the olives into a bowl and enjoy as an appetizer or a salad accompaniment.

TAKE A CHANCE:

• Add 2 or 3 dried red chili peppers.

• Use 1 or 2 teaspoons Harissa Sauce (page 167) instead of cayenne pepper.

In Morocco, olives of every kind are sold on street corners. In this recipe, we mix together green and black olives, then add onion, garlic, and a variety of flavorful herbs and spices. Be forewarned, these flavorful morsels will disappear quickly.

$1/2$ yellow or white onion, coarsely chopped

3 cloves garlic, coarsely chopped

$1/2$ cup fresh lemon juice

$1/4$ cup extra-virgin olive oil

$1/4$ cup chopped fresh cilantro

1 teaspoon paprika

$1/2$ teaspoon ground cumin

$1/4$ teaspoon cayenne pepper

1 cup brine-cured green olives, rinsed

1 cup brine-cured black olives, rinsed

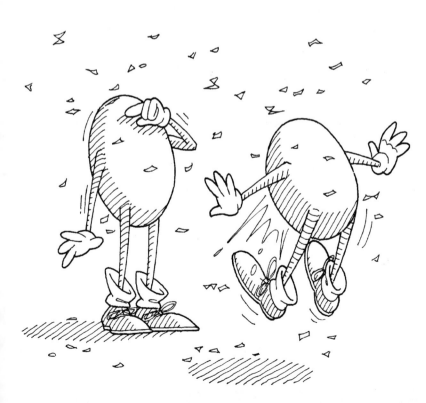

Baked Onion Rings United States

These crunchy, breaded onion rings are a good choice for reducing the fat without giving up the taste in this all-time favorite dish.

4 large yellow or white onions, cut into ¹/₄-inch slices

1 cup bread crumbs

¹/₈ teaspoon ground sage

¹/₈ teaspoon ground rosemary

¹/₈ teaspoon freshly ground black pepper

1 egg

1 tablespoon cold water

YIELD: 6 SERVINGS   PREPARATION TIME: 45 MINUTES

1. Rinse and separate the onion slices under cold water. Drain and pat dry with paper toweling.

2. Mix the bread crumbs, sage, rosemary, and pepper together in a bowl.

3. Lightly beat together the egg and water in a bowl.

4. Dip the onion rings into the egg, then into the bread-crumb mixture, making sure to coat them completely.

5. Lightly spray a baking sheet with a nonstick cooking spray. Arrange the breaded onion rings in a single layer on the sheet. Cover with foil and bake in a 400°F oven for 10 minutes. Uncover and continue to bake for 20 minutes, or until the onion rings are brown and crisp.

6. Serve immediately with Creamy Roasted Garlic Sauce (page 169), or Rouille (page 171).

TAKE A CHANCE:

• Use flavored bread crumbs instead of plain.

• Experiment with different herbs for different flavors.

Roasted Garlic France

1. Remove the papery outer skin from each head of garlic. Do not peel or separate the cloves.

2. Place the garlic in a small baking dish that is just large enough to hold the heads. Drizzle the garlic with the olive oil and dot with the margarine. Cover tightly and bake the garlic in a preheated 350°F oven for 50 minutes, or until the cloves are soft.

3. Remove the skin from the cloves and mash them together. Spread on the bread.

TAKE A CHANCE:

• Add $1/4$ teaspoon dried thyme leaves or herbs de Provence to the olive oil.

• Add 1 tablespoon white wine to the olive oil.

• Omit the olive oil and margarine, and add $3/4$ cup of chicken broth to the baking dish. If necessary add additional broth during cooking. Discard the broth after baking.

• Heads may be wrapped separately in aluminum foil and baked for 1 hour with or without the oil and margarine.

• Serve on pita or sourdough bread.

The savory smell of roasting garlic will permeate every room in the house. If you have been reluctant to try roasted garlic for fear of a strong taste, you will be pleasantly surprised. When garlic is slow-roasted, its cloves are transformed into honey-colored morsels that have a unique mellow sweetness. The soft, caramelized cloves can be added to a variety of dishes or spread on bread in place of butter as shown below.

4 whole heads of garlic

2 teaspoons extra-virgin olive oil

1 teaspoon soy margarine

8 slices toasted French or Italian bread

GARLIC ROASTERS

Terra cotta garlic roasters are almost as easy to find as garlic presses. To use a roaster, follow the instructions for Roasted Garlic above but do not preheat the oven. Just like their big brothers—the clay pot cookers—these roasters are placed in a cold oven. Turn the temperature to 300°F and cook for 30 minutes. Remove the cover and continue to roast an additional 30 minutes, or until the heads turn golden brown.

Garlic roasters can also be used in the microwave. Cook the garlic on full power for 2 to 3 minutes. Although this cooking method is a time saver, the garlic will not brown. So we use the microwave only when we want to add the garlic to a dish for its mellow taste, not when we serve it as a spread.

Cajun Onion Rings United States

There is almost nothing more satisfying than biting into a crisp onion ring. We love the contrasting taste of Cajun spices and sweet onion in this recipe.

4 large sweet onions such as Spanish or Vidalia, peeled and cut into $1/4$-inch slices

2 cups skim milk

$1^1/2$ cups unbleached white flour

$1/2$ teaspoon cayenne pepper

$1/2$ teaspoon dried thyme

$1/8$ teaspoon freshly ground black pepper

2 cups canola oil

YIELD: 6 SERVINGS   PREPARATION TIME: 45 MINUTES

1. Separate the onions into rings and place them in a large bowl along with the milk. Stir well, cover, and set aside for 20 minutes.

2. Place the flour, cayenne pepper, thyme, and black pepper in a medium-sized brown paper bag and mix well.

3. Drain the onions and discard the milk. Place a few rings at a time in the bag, close the bag, and shake well. Remove the onions to a large plate and continue coating the remaining onions.

4. Heat the oil in a deep heavy skillet or a deep fryer for 5 minutes. The temperature of the oil should register 350°F on a deep-frying thermometer. Add the onions a few at a time and cook until golden brown.

5. With a slotted spoon, remove the onions to an ovenproof platter that is lined with paper toweling. Keep the platter in a 200°F oven until all of the onion rings are cooked.

6. Transfer the cooked rings to a serving dish lined with doilies or paper toweling, and serve immediately.

TAKE A CHANCE:

• Add 2 teaspoons chopped fresh parsley to the flour mixture.

SLICING ONIONS

Onions can squirm and wiggle when you're trying to slice them. There are two methods of slicing onions you can use to save yourself a trip to the medicine cabinet:

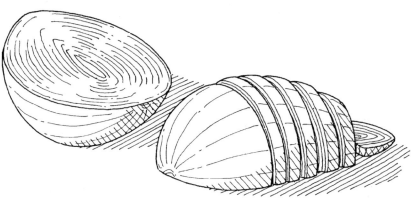

METHOD 1

Cut the onion in half lengthwise. Lay the cut side down on the work surface, and slice the onion either lengthwise or crosswise.

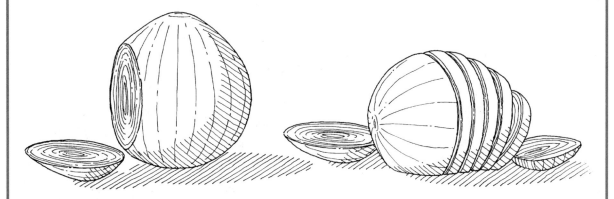

METHOD 2

If you want full slices, stand the onion on one of its ends and slice a small piece from the side. Lay the onion on this cut side (with the piece removed, the onion will stay flat and won't roll) and slice it into full rings.

Giardinera Italy

Enjoy garden-fresh vegetables all year round with this colorful relish.

1 red onion, cut lengthwise into $1/2$-inch slices

3 cloves garlic, cut in half

2 cups cauliflower florets

$1/2$ cup whole small mushrooms, stems removed

1 cup carrots, peeled and cut into $1/4$-inch slices

$1/2$ cup large green olives

1 large sweet red bell pepper, seeded and cut into $1/2$-inch strips

1 cup extra-virgin olive oil

$1/4$ cup cider vinegar

$1/4$ teaspoon dry mustard

6 whole peppercorns

YIELD: 4 SERVINGS   PREPARATION TIME: 24 HOURS

1. Mix all of the ingredients in a large bowl or jar with a tight-fitting lid. Cover and refrigerate at least overnight. One full day will give better flavor.

2. Serve as an appetizer, or use to spice up a tossed salad.

TAKE A CHANCE:

• Add $1/2$ cup Tuscan peppers, drained.

• Use black olives instead of green.

• Don't throw out the marinade after the giardinera is finished. Add a few garlic cloves and some oregano, and use it as a salad dressing.

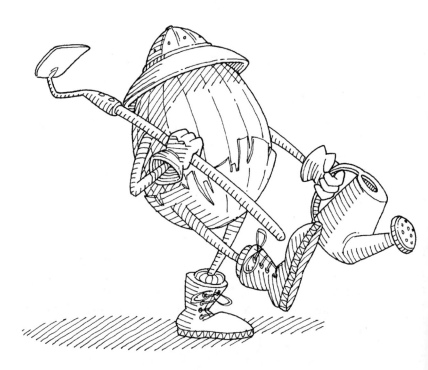

Garlic Mushrooms Spain

A favorite appetizer served at Spanish tapas bars (see below), these sassy garlic mushrooms are a snap to make.

YIELD: 4 SERVINGS   PREPARATION TIME: 20 MINUTES

1. With a sharp knife, cut the stems of the mushrooms evenly with the caps. Leave the mushrooms whole if they are small. Cut the large ones in half or quarters.

2. Place the oil in a large skillet over medium heat. Add the mushrooms and sauté for 1 minute. Add the garlic and sauté another minute. Add the remaining ingredients and sauté 2 minutes more.

3. Transfer the mushrooms and their cooking juice to a serving bowl. Serve immediately with plenty of fresh crusty bread to soak up the wonderful flavorful juices.

TAKE A CHANCE:

- Add the grated zest of 1 lemon.
- Sprinkle the mushrooms with paprika before serving.
- Use 4 finely chopped small dried chili peppers instead of crushed red pepper.

1 pound fresh mushrooms

6 cloves garlic, peeled and thinly sliced lengthwise

3 tablespoons extra-virgin olive oil (preferably Spanish)

$1/4$ cup chicken broth

3 tablespoons fresh lemon juice

2 tablespoons dry sherry (preferably Spanish)

$1/2$ teaspoon crushed red pepper

$1/4$ teaspoon freshly ground black pepper

TAPAS

Originally served in Spanish bars as free snacks, tapas are much like the "happy hour" tidbits served in the United States. Today, in Spain, tapas are enjoyed as snacks as well as appetizers before main meals. More and more Americans are discovering these delectable little bites at tapas bars, which are springing up all over the country.

Tapas range from simple finger foods to more sophisticated morsels. Many prepared foods can be presented as tapas simply by serving them on small dishes along with crackers or bread. On the other hand, many recipes intended as tapas can be served as main dishes by adding a salad, vegetable, or other accompaniment.

Stuffed Mushrooms France

Although the original recipe for these stuffed mushrooms includes ham and pancetta (a rindless bacon), we believe our meatless version is just as tasty.

12 large white mushrooms

2 tablespoons extra-virgin olive oil

2 large shallots, finely chopped

2 cloves garlic, finely chopped

2 tablespoons finely chopped fresh parsley

$1/8$ teaspoon freshly ground black pepper

$1/4$ cup fresh toasted bread crumbs

2 tablespoons finely chopped fresh chives

YIELD: 12 MUSHROOMS   PREPARATION TIME: 40 MINUTES

1. Remove the stems from the mushrooms. Set the caps aside and finely chop the stems.

2. Place 1 tablespoon of the oil in a skillet over medium heat. Add the mushroom caps and sauté for 3 minutes. With a slotted spoon, transfer the caps to a warmed plate.

3. Heat the remaining oil in the skillet. Add the mushroom stems, shallots, garlic, parsley, and black pepper, and sauté for 2 minutes. Add the bread crumbs and sauté another minute.

4. Stuff the mushroom caps with the bread-crumb mixture and place them on a baking sheet that has been lightly coated with nonstick cooking spray. Bake in a 350°F oven for 25 minutes, or until the filling has browned.

5. Garnish with chives and serve immediately.

TAKE A CHANCE:

• Add 1 tablespoon finely chopped walnuts to the filling mixture.

• Omit the chives and garnish with a sprinkling of freshly grated Parmesan cheese.

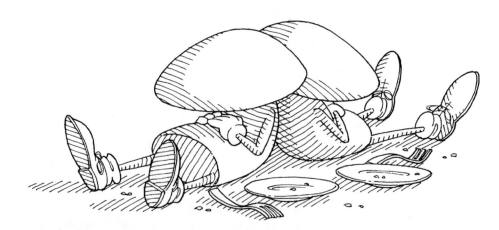

Garlic Shrimp Appetizers Spain

YIELD: 4 SERVINGS   PREPARATION TIME: 2 HOURS

1. Mix all of the ingredients, except the parsley, together in a medium bowl. Cover and marinate in the refrigerator for 1½ hours.

2. With a slotted spoon, transfer the shrimp to a plate and set aside. Place the marinade in a skillet over medium-low heat, and sauté for 1 minute or until the garlic releases its aroma. Remove the garlic and discard.

3. Add the shrimp to the skillet and cook about 2 minutes, or until they just begin to turn pink.

4. Place the shrimp and cooking juices in a decorative bowl. Serve hot.

TAKE A CHANCE:

• Drain the raw marinated shrimp and thread them on metal or wooden skewers. Grill over hot coals until the shrimp turns pink.

• Use white wine instead of sherry.

• Serve the shrimp with Garlic Mayonnaise (page 170) instead of the cooking juices.

These tasty appetizers owe their goodness to the flavorful combination of garlic, sherry, and olive oil. Double the recipe and serve over rice for an easy dinner entrée.

1 pound medium shrimp, cleaned

6 cloves garlic, sliced

½ cup dry sherry (preferably Spanish)

3 tablespoons extra-virgin olive oil (preferably Spanish)

1 tablespoon finely chopped fresh parsley

Spicy Ceviche Mexico

The lime juice actually cooks the fish in this seafood cocktail, but the onion, garlic, and chili peppers give it its spicy flavor.

1 1/2 pounds fish fillets such as bass, sole, or red snapper, cut into 1/2-inch cubes

8 ounces small scallops

1 cup finely chopped yellow or white onion

2 cloves garlic, coarsely chopped

3 serrano chili peppers, seeded and finely chopped

1 1/2 cups lime juice

1/4 cup finely chopped fresh cilantro

1/4 teaspoon freshly ground black pepper

YIELD: 4 SERVINGS   PREPARATION TIME: 3 HOURS

1. Mix all of the ingredients in a shallow glass bowl. If necessary, add more lime juice to cover the fish completely. Cover the bowl and marinate the fish for 2 1/2 hours in the refrigerator.

2. Discard the garlic and serve immediately.

TAKE A CHANCE:

• Add one or more of the following: 1 to 2 whole seeded and diced tomatoes, 1/4 teaspoon hot sauce, 3 tablespoons extra-virgin olive oil.

• Reduce the amount of fish fillets to 1 pound and add 8 ounces of shelled, deveined small shrimp. The shrimp should be cooked and added to the marinade shortly before serving.

• Use fresh lemon juice instead of lime, or a mixture of both.

Trivia Tidbit

For a more subtle garlic flavoring in any recipe, substitute elephant garlic for the regular variety.

Marinated White Fish South Africa

YIELD: 4 SERVINGS   PREPARATION TIME: 2 1/2 HOURS

1. Place $^1/_2$ cup of the water and $1^1/_2$ teaspoons of the lemon juice in a medium skillet over high heat. Bring to a boil and add the peppercorns and fish. Reduce the heat to medium-low and simmer for 3 minutes, or until the fish flakes when tested with a fork.

2. Using a slotted spoon, remove the fish from the pan and place in a bowl. Discard the cooking liquid.

3. Place the oil in a small saucepan over medium heat. Add the onion and sauté for 2 minutes. Add the flour and stir constantly until it is absorbed. Continue to stir while gradually adding the vinegar and the remaining water and lemon juice. Add the sugar and black pepper, and continue to stir until the sugar is dissolved.

4. Pour the sauce over the fish and mix well. Cover and refrigerate for 2 hours.

5. Place the chilled fish on a platter and garnish with parsley before serving.

TAKE A CHANCE:

• Add $^1/_8$ teaspoon crushed red pepper to the fish as it cooks.

• Add $^1/_8$ teaspoon cumin to the sauce as it cooks.

Unlike its Mexican cousin, Spicy Ceviche (page 32), this pickled fish is not very hot, and it is cooked before it is marinated.

1 pound flounder or cod fillets, cut in 2-inch cubes

1 cup water

3 tablespoons fresh lemon juice

6 whole peppercorns

3 teaspoons canola oil

1 onion, thinly sliced

1 teaspoon unbleached white flour

$1^1/_2$ teaspoons cider vinegar

1 teaspoon date sugar

$^1/_8$ teaspoon freshly ground black pepper

2 teaspoons chopped fresh parsley

Baccala Italy

*B*accala, a popular garlic-laden codfish appetizer, is one dish for which there are many regional Mediterranean versions. The cod must be soaked at least 24 hours before preparing this dish.

2 pounds dried salted cod

8 cloves garlic, minced

3/4 cup fresh lemon juice

1 tablespoon capers

1 large lemon cut into wedges

YIELD: 6 SERVINGS   PREPARATION TIME: 1 1/2 DAYS

1. Put the cod in a large mixing bowl and cover with water. Cover the bowl with aluminum foil and let the fish soak in the refrigerator for 24 hours. Change the water every 4 to 8 hours to remove the excess salt.

2. Transfer the fish to a cutting board. With your fingers or a fork, flake the cod and remove the bones and scales. Place the flaked fish on a large, flat platter.

3. Mix together the garlic, lemon juice, and capers in a small bowl. Pour this marinade over the flaked fish and mix thoroughly. The mixture should be very wet. If it is too dry, add more lemon juice. Cover and refrigerate for at least 3 hours.

4. Mix thoroughly, garnish with lemon wedges, and serve.

TAKE A CHANCE:

• Add 1/2 teaspoon crushed red pepper to the marinade mixture.

Trivia Tidbit

It is believed that Marco Polo discovered the garlic clove during his travels to the Orient and brought it back to Italy. From Italy, garlic's popularity spread through the entire Mediterranean region, where it became a common ingredient in a wide variety of dishes.

Bacalao Spain

YIELD: 6 SERVINGS PREPARATION TIME: 1 ½ DAYS

1. Put the cod in a large mixing bowl and cover with water. Cover the bowl with aluminum foil and let the fish soak in the refrigerator for 24 hours. Change the water every 4 to 8 hours to remove the excess salt.

2. Transfer the fish to a cutting board. With your fingers or a fork, flake the cod and remove the bones and scales. Place the flaked fish on a platter and set aside.

3. Place the garlic and 1 tablespoon of the oil in a small saucepan over very low heat. Slow-cook the garlic until it is soft but not brown, about 15 minutes. Using a slotted spoon, remove the garlic to a small bowl and set aside.

4. Heat the remaining oil in a large skillet. Add the cod and sauté for 5 to 10 minutes or until the fish is golden brown. Add the garlic to the pan and continue to sauté another minute.

5. Transfer the fish to a platter and serve immediately.

TAKE A CHANCE:

• Add a small seeded and chopped tomato to the skillet when cooking the fish.

• Mix the sautéed fish with Garlic Mayonnaise (page 170).

*T*he Spanish commonly serve this salted cod appetizer in tapas bars (page 29). Similar to Italian Baccala (page 34), Bacalao calls for olive oil instead of lemon juice, giving it a completely different taste. Look for Spanish olive oil, which has a light, fruity flavor. Like baccala, the dried salted cod must be soaked at least 24 hours before preparing this dish.

2 pounds dried salted cod

10 cloves garlic, coarsely chopped

4 tablespoons extra-virgin olive oil (preferably Spanish)

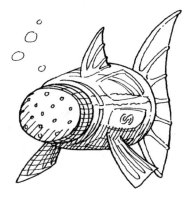

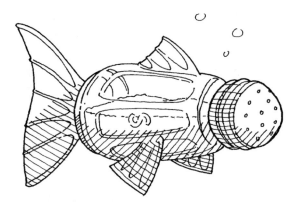

Egg Rolls with Garlic Sauce Philippines

Filipino egg rolls, called lumpia, are double-wrapped—first in lettuce, then in a freshly made wrapper. The egg roll is then dipped into a wonderful garlic-filled sauce.

Wrappers

1 cup unbleached flour

1 cup water

1 egg, lightly beaten

Sauce

1 1/2 cups water

1/4 cup shoyu or tamari soy sauce

1/4 cup date sugar

1/4 cup arrowroot

6 cloves garlic, crushed

Filling

1 yellow or white onion, finely chopped

1 tablespoon canola oil

2 cloves garlic, crushed

8 ounces small shrimp, cleaned and cut into small pieces

1/2 cup bamboo shoots

YIELD: 8 EGG ROLLS   PREPARATION TIME: 1 HOUR

1. To make the wrappers, mix the flour and water together in a bowl. Add the egg and stir until the batter is smooth. Spray an 8-inch skillet with nonstick cooking spray and place over medium heat. When the skillet is hot, spoon 1/4 cup of batter into the skillet and rotate the pan until the batter covers the bottom. Cook 2 to 3 minutes—when the wrapper is fully cooked, it will begin to curl away from the edges of the pan and will easily lift out with a spatula. Repeat the process with the remaining batter (should yield 8 wrappers). Stack the wrappers on a plate and separate with paper towels.

2. To make the sauce, place the water, shoyu, and sugar in a small saucepan and heat almost to boiling. Reduce the heat to medium and gradually add the arrowroot, stirring constantly for 3 to 4 minutes or until the sauce begins to thicken. Remove the pan from the heat and let cool for 20 minutes. Stir the garlic into the cooled sauce.

3. To make the filling, place the oil in a large skillet over medium heat, add the onion, and sauté for 2 minutes. Add the garlic and shrimp, and sauté another minute. Add the bamboo shoots and black pepper, and cook another 5 minutes. Drain any liquid from the pan.

4. To assemble the egg rolls, lay a wrapper on a work surface and place a lettuce leaf on top. Spoon about 1 1/2 tablespoons of the filling on the lettuce. Bring the right and left sides of the wrapper over the filling, then roll up the wrapper from the bottom. Place the roll, seam side down, on a serving plate. Repeat with the remaining wrappers and filling.

5. Pour the sauce into a bowl and serve alongside the egg rolls.

- Add $1/2$ cup diced water chestnuts to the filling. Cook along with the bamboo shoots.

- Use 8 ounces finely chopped chicken instead of shrimp.

$1/4$ teaspoon freshly ground black pepper

8 lettuce leaves

Rolled Tortillas Mexico / United States

YIELD: 4 SERVINGS PREPARATION TIME: 1$1/4$ HOURS

1. Place the tortillas on a cutting board and spread 2 tablespoons of cream cheese on each. Evenly sprinkle the onions, tomatoes, and cilantro on top.

2. Fold the left and right sides of each tortilla to the center (about $1/2$ inch), then roll them up from the bottom. Cover with plastic wrap and refrigerate 1 hour.

3. Using a sharp knife. Cut the chilled tortillas into 1-inch slices. Arrange the slices on a plate and serve with Salsa Cruda.

TAKE A CHANCE:

- Use finely chopped white onion or scallions instead of pickled onions.

- Add $1/2$ teaspoon finely minced jalapeño pepper to the filling.

- Serve with nonfat sour cream instead of salsa.

Although tortillas, pickled onions, and salsa are staples of Mexican cuisine, you won't find anything on any menu that combines them quite like this appetizer does.

2 medium-sized flour tortillas

4 tablespoons nonfat cream cheese

2 tablespoons finely chopped Lime-Marinated Onion Rings (page 157)

2 tablespoons seeded, finely chopped tomatoes

2 teaspoons finely chopped fresh cilantro

$1/4$ cup Salsa Cruda (page 22)

Tiny Chicken Turnovers Cuba

Although traditionally these Cuban turnovers are made with ground beef, we experimented with ground chicken and found them to be just as delicious. Another great thing about these tasty tidbits is that they can be prepared ahead of time.

1 egg white, lightly beaten

1 cup Salsa Cruda (page 22)

Dough

2 cups unbleached white flour

1 teaspoon baking powder

$1/2$ cup soy margarine, chilled and cut into small pieces

$1/4$ cup cold water

Filling

1 pound lean, ground free-range chicken

1 tablespoon canola oil

1 yellow or white onion, finely chopped

2 cloves garlic, crushed

$1/2$ teaspoon chili powder

1 teaspoon finely chopped fresh cilantro

$1/4$ teaspoon freshly ground black pepper

YIELD: 12 TURNOVERS   PREPARATION TIME: 1 $1/2$ HOURS

1. To make the dough, combine the flour and baking powder in a large bowl. Add the margarine and blend with a fork or pastry blender until it resembles coarse meal. Add just enough cold water to hold the mixture together. Gather the dough into a ball and knead once. Wrap the dough in plastic and chill for 1 hour.

2. To make the filling, heat the oil in a large skillet, add the onion, and sauté 2 minutes. Add the garlic and chili powder, and sauté another minute. Add the chicken, cilantro, and black pepper, and sauté until the chicken is no longer pink.

3. To assemble the turnovers, place the chilled dough on a floured board and roll it out to $1/8$-inch thickness. Cut the dough into twelve 4-inch squares. Put 1 heaping tablespoon of filling in the middle of each square, then fold the dough in half to form a triangle. Lightly pinch the edges together to seal.

4. Arrange the turnovers on a baking sheet that has been lightly coated with cooking spray. Brush the tops of the turnovers with the egg white, and bake in a 400°F oven for 25 minutes, or until golden brown.

5. Serve immediately with Salsa Cruda.

TAKE A CHANCE:

• Use whole wheat flour for the dough.

• Use cayenne pepper instead of chili powder.

• Add 3 seeded, chopped jalapeño peppers to the filling.

Pickled Herring Russia / Scandinavia

YIELD: 1 QUART PREPARATION TIME: 2 DAYS

1. Place the herring in a large bowl with enough fresh water to cover. Cover the bowl and refrigerate for 6 to 8 hours.

2. Debone the herring, then cut it into bite-sized pieces. Alternate layers of herring and onions in a heatproof quart jar. Fill the jar almost to the top.

3. Mix the boiling water with the vinegar, then pour it into the jar. Add the oil and seal the jar tightly. Refrigerate for at least 1 day.

4. Before serving, shake the jar well. Spoon the pickled herring and onion slices into a serving bowl, and enjoy with crackers or black bread.

TAKE A CHANCE:

• Add 1 cup sliced mushrooms to the jar.

The briny tartness of this dish is enjoyed throughout northern Europe. Use only smaltzer herring, which come in barrels of brine and are found in many gourmet shops and delis.

2 smaltzer herring

3 yellow or white onions, thinly sliced

3 cups boiling water

3 tablespoons distilled white vinegar

1 tablespoon oil

ROASTING PEPPERS

Roasting peppers is easy, and it gives all types of peppers—from the mild bell to the fiery chili—a mellow, smoky flavor. Roasting also frees the pepper of its tough transparent skin. When handling hot chili peppers and when roasting peppers of any kind, we recommend wearing rubber gloves because the pepper oil can burn your skin.

There are several methods used to roast peppers. No matter which method you use, first make a small cut in the pepper near its stem. This will allow the steam to escape during cooking. If you have a gas stove, large peppers can be held with tongs over a medium flame until they begin to blister, or they can be set right on the burner. Frequently turn the peppers to char them evenly. Place the hot, charred peppers in a paper bag. Seal the bag and allow the peppers to cool. When they are cool enough to handle, peel off the skin under cold running water. The roasted peppers can be used immediately or frozen for later use.

Peppers can also be roasted on a barbecue grill or under the broiler. Small peppers, however, must be cooked in a pan.

Vegetable Hoagies Italy

Whether you know them as hoagies, heroes, submarines, or grinders, these sandwiches can be cut and served as appetizers. Our version of this sandwich is is a veritable vegetable feast.

6 cloves garlic, crushed

1/4 cup fresh lemon juice

2 tablespoons extra-virgin olive oil

1/4 teaspoon dried oregano

1/8 teaspoon freshly ground black pepper

4 Italian-bread rolls, about 6 inches long

1 yellow or white onion, cut into paper-thin slices

1 tomato, seeded and chopped

2 zucchini, thinly sliced

12 white mushrooms, trimmed and thinly sliced

12 pitted, black olives

12 slices provolone cheese

2 roasted red bell peppers, cut into 1/2-inch strips

6 Tuscan peppers, chopped

1 cup shredded lettuce

1. In a small bowl, mix together the garlic, lemon juice, olive oil, oregano, and black pepper. Toss in the onion, tomato, zucchini, mushrooms, and olives, and mix well. Set aside and allow the vegetables to marinate.

2. Cut the rolls lengthwise but not all the way through. Using a spoon spread some of the marinade mixture on the inside of the bread.

3. Place 3 slices of provolone cheese on each roll, and spoon the vegetable mixture on top. Top with the roasted peppers, Tuscan peppers and lettuce. Drizzle any leftover marinade over the lettuce.

4. Close the sandwiches and eat as is, or cut them into small pieces and serve as appetizers.

TAKE A CHANCE:

• Use mozzarella cheese either with or instead of the provolone.

• Add 1 teaspoon wine vinegar to the oil.

• Use a roasted red chili pepper instead of the bell pepper.

Chapter 3

Succulent Salad Sensations

Fortunately, not all salads have to be green, although the leafy kinds are always fun, especially when dressed up with onions and garlic. The robust flavors of alliums add sparkle, flavor, and nutrition to salads of all sorts. In this chapter, we present a wide variety of our favorites—some leafy, others, not so.

Cabbage Salad with Peppered Onions Vietnam

*T*his hearty salad can become addictive. Luckily, it is very easy to make.

1 small cabbage, thinly sliced

1 large carrot, shredded

2 Thai chili peppers, finely chopped

3 tablespoons coarsely chopped fresh mint

3 tablespoons coarsely chopped fresh cilantro

3 tablespoons crushed unsalted peanuts

Dressing

1 white onion, cut lengthwise into thin slices

3 cloves garlic, thinly sliced

$1/4$ cup white vinegar

2 teaspoons vegetable oil

$1/2$ teaspoon freshly ground black pepper

Accompaniment

$1/2$ cup fish sauce (nuoc mam)*

2 teaspoons Garlic Chili Paste (page 169)

* Available in Asian grocery stores.

YIELD: 4 SERVINGS   PREPARATION TIME: 20 MINUTES

1. Combine the dressing ingredients in a small bowl and allow to set at least 20 minutes. Stir occasionally.

2. In another small bowl, mix together the fish sauce and Garlic Chili Paste. Set aside.

3. Toss the cabbage, carrot, chili peppers, mint, and cilantro in a large bowl. Add the dressing and toss again.

4. Garnish with peanuts and serve with extra fish sauce on the side.

TAKE A CHANCE:

• To reduce the tartness of the dressing, add $1/4$ teaspoon sugar.

• For a hearty salad, add 1 cup cooked, shredded chicken.

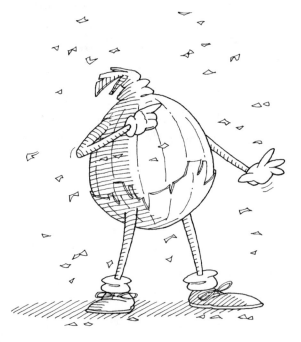

Caesar Salad Mexico / United States

1. Combine the garlic, lime juice, and olive oil in a large bowl. Mix well and let sit for 15 minutes.

2. Add the anchovies, dry mustard, Worcestershire sauce, and black pepper to the bowl, and mix well. Add the egg and stir well, making sure to coat the sides of the bowl with the dressing.

3. Add the lettuce and toss until the leaves are thoroughly coated with dressing. Sprinkle with cheese and toss again.

4. Garnish with Garlic Croutons and serve immediately.

TAKE A CHANCE:

• Make the salad in a wooden bowl. Peel the garlic and cut each clove in half. Rub the garlic around the insides of the bowl. The used cloves can then be discarded or added to the salad.

• All right, so you won't try the anchovies. No problem, just skip them. But don't skip over this recipe.

• Use fresh lemon juice instead of lime.

• Top with shrimp, scallops, or sliced grilled chicken.

Although a staple in the United States, this salad was actually invented by two Italian brothers for their restaurant in Tijuana, Mexico. Some Caesar salad enthusiasts believe the garlic cloves should be rubbed around the insides of a wooden salad bowl, giving the salad a gentle garlic flavor. But for true garlic lovers, lots of finely minced or crushed garlic tossed into the salad is the only way to go.

4 cloves garlic, finely chopped or crushed

1/4 cup fresh lime juice

1/4 cup extra-virgin olive oil

8 anchovy fillets, mashed

1/4 teaspoon dry mustard

1/2 teaspoon Worcestershire sauce

1/4 teaspoon freshly ground black pepper

1 egg, lightly beaten

1 head romaine lettuce, torn into pieces

1/4 cup freshly grated Romano cheese

1 cup Garlic Croutons (page 158)

Garlicky Broccoli Salad Italy

This wonderful salad contains two of our all-time favorite tastes—garlic and lemon.

1 pound fresh broccoli, peeled and coarsely chopped

8 cloves garlic, finely minced

1 cup fresh lemon juice

YIELD: 4 SERVINGS   PREPARATION TIME: 3 1/2 HOURS

1. Combine the garlic and lemon juice in a small bowl and set aside for 15 minutes.

2. Steam the broccoli for 3 minutes. It should still be bright green and crisp.

3. Arrange the broccoli on a flat plate and pour the garlic-lemon marinade on top. Cover and refrigerate for at least 3 hours, turning the broccoli several times to marinate evenly.

4. Mix well before serving.

TAKE A CHANCE:

• Sprinkle with crushed red pepper before serving.

• Cut the broccoli into 3-inch pieces instead of chopping it.

Antipasto Italy

This salad can be made large for a crowd or small for an individual serving, but it is always just right with crunchy onions and a garlicky dressing.

2 cups romaine lettuce, torn into pieces

2 cups red or green leaf lettuce, torn into pieces

2 cucumbers, seeded and cut into 4-inch spears

YIELD: 4 SERVINGS   PREPARATION TIME: 30 MINUTES

1. Mix the dressing ingredients together in a small bowl. Allow to stand for 10 minutes.

2. Place the lettuce on a serving platter, and arrange all of the remaining ingredients, except the grated cheese and Scallion Paint Brushes, on top.

3. Stir the dressing well and drizzle it over the vegetables. Garnish with the grated cheese and Scallion Paint Brushes. Serve immediately.

TAKE A CHANCE:

- Use a Vidalia onion or Lime-Marinated Onion Rings (page 157) instead of the red onion.
- Garnish the platter with wedges of hard boiled egg.
- Add $1/2$ cup sliced mushrooms or carrots.
- Add $1/2$ teaspoon crushed red pepper to the dressing.
- Use Creamy Roasted Garlic Sauce (page 169) or Red Onion Vinaigrette (page 160) as a dressing.

PEELING GARLIC

To separate the cloves from a head of garlic, first set the head on a counter. Place your palm or the flat surface of a large knife on top of the head and press down. The cloves will separate like flower petals.

To peel the skin from an individual clove, place the clove on a counter and press down on it with the flat side of a large knife. Or you can hit the side of the knife with the palm of your hand. This will loosen the skin for easy removal. Be sure to remove the hard knob at the end of the clove before using.

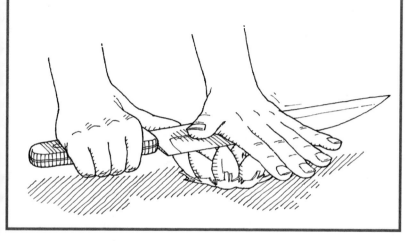

2 tomatoes, cut into wedges and seeded

16 asparagus stalks, steamed and cooled to room temperature

8 marinated artichoke hearts

1 medium sweet red bell pepper, sliced

1 medium red onion, cut lengthwise into 1-inch slices

$1/2$ cup pitted brine-cured black olives

8 Tuscan peppers

6 slices mozzarella cheese

1 tablespoon freshly grated Parmesan or Romano cheese

4 Scallion Paint Brushes (page 176)

Dressing

3 cloves garlic, crushed

$1/4$ cup extra-virgin olive oil

$1/4$ cup fresh lemon juice

2 teaspoons chopped fresh oregano, or 1 teaspoon dried

2 teaspoons finely chopped fresh Italian parsley

$1/4$ teaspoon freshly ground black pepper

Lentil Salad Southern Europe / Greece / Turkey

*L*entils are eaten extensively throughout the Mediterranean. This salad has a fresh exotic taste and lots of garlic and green onions.

2 cups lentils, rinsed and drained

3 tablespoons extra-virgin olive oil

3 cloves garlic, minced

3 scallions, coarsely chopped

1 teaspoon ground cumin

$1/2$ cup lemon juice

$1/8$ teaspoon freshly ground black pepper

YIELD: 4 SERVINGS   PREPARATION TIME: 1 HOUR

1. Place the lentils in a medium saucepan with enough water to cover. Bring to a boil, then simmer for 20 minutes or until the lentils are tender. Drain and cool.

2. Place 2 tablespoons of the oil in a large saucepan over medium heat. Add the garlic, scallions, and cumin, and sauté for 1 minute.

3. Transfer the lentils to a serving bowl, add the lemon juice, black pepper, and the garlic–scallion mixture. Mix well. Cover and let sit for 30 minutes.

4. Before serving, stir the lentils well and drizzle with the remaining oil.

TAKE A CHANCE:

• Add a large seeded and chopped tomato to the ingredients in step 3.

• Add 2 teaspoons fresh chopped parsley.

• Use cayenne pepper instead of cumin.

• Garnish with a chopped hard boiled egg.

Tomato Salad Germany / Italy

YIELD: 4 SERVINGS   PREPARATION TIME: 1¼ HOURS

1. Place the onion, garlic, basil, oil, and black pepper in a large bowl. Mix well. Add the tomatoes and stir to coat. Cover the bowl and refrigerate for 1 hour.

2. Stir before serving.

TAKE A CHANCE:

• Use cilantro, mint, or oregano instead of basil.

• Add a diced fresh chili pepper.

• Add a seeded, coarsely chopped cucumber.

• Add a seeded green bell pepper that is cut into 1-inch pieces.

European explorers brought garlic and onions to the New World and returned home with tomatoes. This salad, which pairs these ingredients of the Old and New World, is popular among the Germans and Italians. Be sure to enjoy this salad with some crusty bread. You'll need it to scoop up every juicy mouthful.

1 yellow or white onion, thinly sliced

2 cloves garlic, crushed

3 large basil leaves, cut into strips

3 tablespoons extra-virgin olive oil

¼ teaspoon freshly ground black pepper

4 large tomatoes, cut into eighths

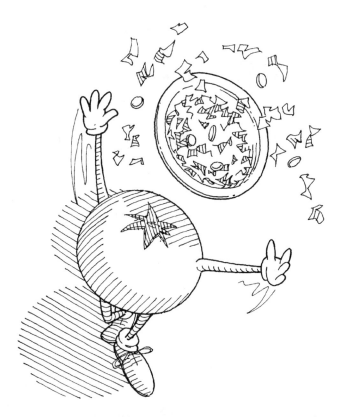

Crunchy Cucumber Salad India

Cucumbers, which are native to northwest India, are paired with garlic and onions in this delicious salad.

1 clove garlic, finely chopped

2 scallions, thinly sliced

3 tablespoons extra-virgin olive oil

1 tablespoon balsamic vinegar

1/2 teaspoon cumin seeds

2 cucumbers, peeled and thinly sliced

YIELD: 4 SERVINGS   PREPARATION TIME: 1 1/2 HOURS

1. Mix all of the ingredients, except the cucumbers, together in a medium bowl. Add the cucumbers and toss to coat. Cover the bowl and refrigerate at least 1 hour.

2. Toss the cucumbers and serve.

TAKE A CHANCE:

• Use 2 coarsely chopped shallots or 1/4 cup thinly sliced yellow or white onion instead of the scallions.

• Use lemon juice instead of balsamic vinegar.

• Garnish with 2 tablespoons chopped cilantro before serving.

Beet Salad Russia

Beets and onions are popular root vegetables in Russia. Here they are paired together in a refreshing salad.

4 fresh beets, peeled, cooked, and thinly sliced

1/2 cup thinly sliced yellow or white onion

1/4 cup canola oil

2 tablespoons distilled white vinegar

1/4 teaspoon black pepper

YIELD: 4 SERVINGS   PREPARATION TIME: 1 HOUR

1. Place all of the ingredients in a medium bowl and mix well. Cover and refrigerate for at least 1 hour.

2. Toss the beets and onions before serving.

TAKE A CHANCE:

• Use 2 finely chopped scallions instead of onion.

• Add 1/2 teaspoon grated orange rind to the ingredients.

• Use balsamic vinegar instead of white vinegar.

Black Bean Salad Latin America / United States

YIELD: 4 SERVINGS   PREPARATION TIME: 1½ HOURS

1. Mix all of the dressing ingredients together in a large bowl. Add the black beans, tomatoes, onion, and jalapeño pepper, and toss to coat. Cover the bowl and refrigerate for 1 hour.

2. Before serving, toss the salad well and garnish with scallions.

TAKE A CHANCE:

• Use pinto beans or rice instead of black beans.

• Garnish with ¼ cup chopped red onion instead of scallions.

• Use ¼ teaspoon crushed red pepper instead of jalapeño pepper.

Trivia Tidbit

Crushed garlic can be applied to the skin to lessen the sting of a scorpion. Bee sting victims can apply a thick slice of onion to the affected area.

---

*B*lack beans are used extensively in many Latin cultures. With the rising popularity of Southwestern cooking, black beans are finally catching on in the United States.

3 cups cooked black beans

2 tomatoes, seeded and diced

½ cup sliced yellow or white onion

1 jalapeño pepper, finely chopped

2 scallions, finely chopped

Dressing

3 cloves garlic, finely chopped

3 tablespoons extra-virgin olive oil

3 tablespoons white wine vinegar

½ teaspoon chili powder

¼ teaspoon cayenne pepper

½ teaspoon freshly ground black pepper

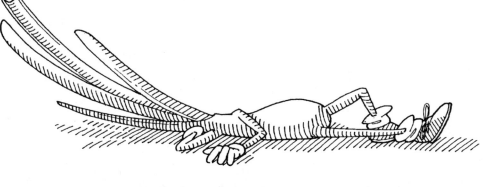

Pasta Tabbouleh Lebanon

We love the fresh taste of tabbouleh. Here, we've traded the traditional bulgar wheat for small pasta shells.

3 cups cooked small pasta shells

2 scallions, finely chopped

2 large tomatoes, seeded and coarsely chopped

1 large cucumber, seeded and coarsely chopped

1/4 cup finely chopped fresh cilantro

1/2 cup finely chopped fresh mint

Dressing

1/4 cup fresh lemon juice

3 tablespoons extra-virgin olive oil

3 cloves garlic, finely minced

1/8 teaspoon freshly ground black pepper

YIELD: 4 SERVING   PREPARATION TIME: 1 1/4 HOURS

1. Mix all of the dressing ingredients together in a small bowl.

2. Place all of the remaining ingredients, except the mint, in a large bowl and toss. Add the dressing and mix well. Cover the bowl and refrigerate 1 hour.

3. Before serving, toss the salad well and garnish with mint.

TAKE A CHANCE:

• Use 2 finely chopped shallots instead of scallions.

• Use bulgar wheat instead of pasta.

• Use fresh basil instead of mint.

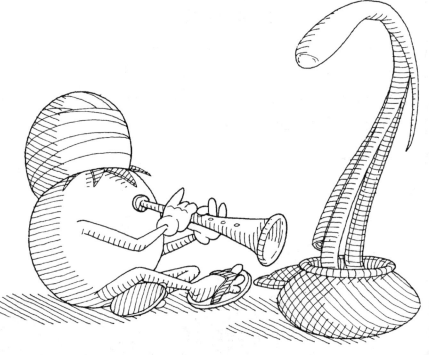

Red Cabbage Salad Denmark

1. Mix together the dressing ingredients in a small bowl.

2. Place the cabbage, apples, and onion in a large bowl, add the dressing, and toss well.

3. Serve immediately.

TAKE A CHANCE:

• Add 1 tablespoon crushed caraway seeds to the dressing.

Sweet apples play off the tart onions and dressing in this simple salad.

1 1/2 cups shredded red cabbage

2 apples, coarsely grated

1 yellow or white onion, coarsely chopped

Dressing

2 tablespoons canola oil

1 tablespoon red wine vinegar

2 cloves garlic, crushed

Yam Salad South Africa

1. Place all of the ingredients in a large bowl and mix well. Cover the bowl and refrigerate 1 hour.

2. Toss well before serving.

TAKE A CHANCE:

• Use sweet potatoes instead of yams.

• Use yellow bell pepper instead of green.

This crunchy, colorful salad makes great picnic fare.

4 yams, cooked, and cubed

1/2 cup sliced yellow or white onion

1/2 cup diced green pepper

1/4 cup diced celery

3 tablespoons fresh lemon juice

2 teaspoons canola oil

1/8 teaspoon freshly ground black pepper

Spicy Orange & Onion Salad Turkey

*A*n unlikely combination, this
refreshing salad is easy to
prepare.

2 tablespoons canola oil

3 tablespoons fresh lemon
juice

1/8 teaspoon freshly ground
black pepper

4 navel oranges, peeled and
thinly sliced crosswise

1 red onion, thinly sliced

12 brine-cured black olives

1/4 cup fresh mint leaves

YIELD: 4 SERVINGS   PREPARATION TIME: 1 HOUR

1. Mix together the oil, lemon juice, and black pepper in a large
bowl. Add the oranges, onion, and olives, and mix well. Cover
the bowl and refrigerate 30 minutes.

2. Mix the salad, garnish with mint, and serve.

TAKE A CHANCE:

• Use shallots instead of red onion.

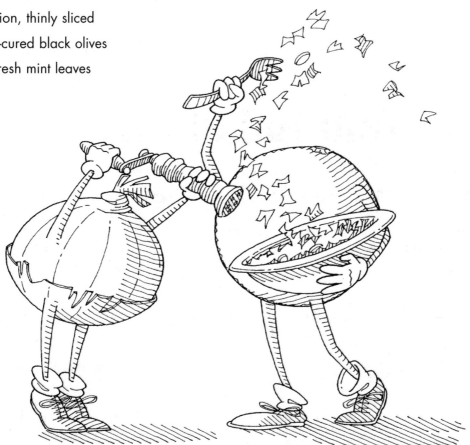

Eggplant Caponata Italy

Sautéed eggplant crunchy with bits of celery and chopped onions makes a delicious salad or appetizer.

YIELD: 4 SERVINGS   PREPARATION TIME: 45 MINUTES

1. Place the broth in a large skillet over medium-low heat. Add the eggplant and sauté until soft, about 10 minutes. With a slotted spoon, transfer the eggplant to a bowl, cover, and set aside.

2. Place the oil and onion in the skillet, and sauté over low heat until the onion begins to caramelize, about 15 minutes. With a slotted spoon, transfer the onions to the bowl with the eggplant.

3. Add the celery to the skillet, and sauté it until it begins to soften, about 2 minutes. (If the pan is dry, add another 2 tablespoons of broth or oil.)

4. Return all of the vegetables to the skillet. Add the tomato paste, capers, vinegar, and cayenne pepper, and stir well. Cook for 10 minutes or until all of the ingredients are well-combined.

5. Serve immediately with crackers or pita bread.

TAKE A CHANCE:

• Add $1/4$ cup chopped green bell pepper.

• Use paprika instead of cayenne pepper.

• Serve along with Bruschetta (page 188).

$1/4$ cup Vegetable Broth (page 59)

1 eggplant, peeled and cut into $1/4$-inch pieces

2 tablespoons extra-virgin olive oil

1 yellow or white onion, chopped

1 celery rib, trimmed and chopped

2 teaspoons tomato paste

1 tablespoon capers

2 teaspoons red wine vinegar

$1/8$ teaspoon cayenne pepper

Spicy Mashed Potato Salad Peru

*N*ew World potatoes and chili peppers are mixed with Old World onions and lemon in this very different version of potato salad. While the original recipe blends the potatoes until smooth, we like to leave it somewhat chunky.

4 potatoes, boiled and drained

1 yellow or white onion, finely chopped

3/4 cup fresh lemon juice

1 teaspoon chili powder

2 tablespoons olive oil

3 jalapeño chili peppers, seeded and finely chopped

2 tablespoons chopped cilantro

YIELD: 4 SERVINGS   PREPARATION TIME: 30 MINUTES

1. Place the potatoes, onion, lemon juice, chili powder, and oil in a food processor. Process to the desired consistency. Add more lemon juice or oil if necessary.

2. Transfer the potatoes to a serving bowl and stir in the chili peppers. Garnish with cilantro and serve immediately.

TAKE A CHANCE:

• Add 1 teaspoon crushed elephant garlic

• Garnish with finely chopped chili peppers instead of cilantro.

• Use leeks instead of onion.

• Use Vegetable Broth (page 59) instead of lemon juice.

Trivia Tidbit

It isn't always necessary to peel potatoes before mashing them. Potato skin contains a number of vitamins. Leaving the skin on also gives the dish character and a little color. Try it!

Kim Chee Korea

YIELD: 4 SERVINGS   PREPARATION TIME: 2 TO 3 DAYS

1. Place the cabbage in a glass or ceramic bowl. Sprinkle with salt and let stand about 4 hours or until the cabbage wilts. Rinse and drain. Add all of the remaining ingredients, except the sesame oil, and mix well.

2. Transfer the cabbage into sterilized jars, cover tightly, and store in a cool place for 2 days.

3. If the kim chee is not pickled enough for your taste, replace the lid and store another day or two.

4. Serve with the sesame oil, which can be drizzled on the cabbage at the table.

TAKE A CHANCE:

• To turn up the heat, add more chili peppers or cayenne pepper to taste.

Spicy hot and full of garlic, this cabbage salad is served with almost every meal in Korea. Traditionally, freshly made kim chee is placed in large jars and buried for many months to mature. Our version is ready in 2 to 3 days, depending on your taste. Be sure to use a jar with a tight-fitting lid as kim chee gives off a pungent odor that can permeate your refrigerator.

2 pounds Napa cabbage, coarsely chopped

2 teaspoons sea salt

6 scallions, coarsely chopped

10 cloves garlic, finely chopped

2 teaspoons finely chopped fresh ginger

2 teaspoons chili powder

4 serrano chili peppers, seeded and finely chopped

1 teaspoon Sucanat

$1/4$ cup shoyu or tamari soy sauce

$1/4$ cup water

$1/2$ cup distilled white vinegar

$1/4$ cup light sesame oil

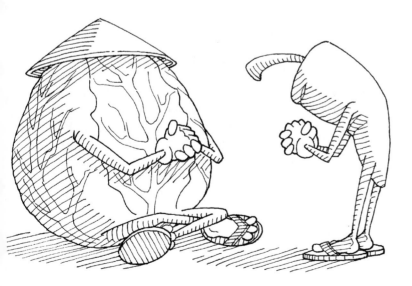

Poached Chicken Salad Aioli France

The herbs de Provence add a touch of the French hillside to this delightful salad.

4 boneless free-range chicken breasts

1/4 cup shredded carrot

1/4 cup diced celery

1/4 teaspoon herbs de Provence

1/4 cup Garlic Mayonnaise (page 170)

1/8 teaspoon freshly ground black pepper

2 tablespoons finely chopped fresh parsley

YIELD: 4 SERVINGS   PREPARATION TIME: 1 1/2 HOURS

1. Place the chicken in a medium saucepan and cover with water. Bring to a boil, reduce the heat to medium, and simmer the chicken for 10 minutes, or until it is just cooked. Transfer the chicken to a plate, cover, and cool for 15 minutes.

2. Shred the chicken and place it in a bowl. Add the remaining ingredients and mix well. Cover the bowl and refrigerate for 1 hour.

3. Before serving, mix well and garnish with parsley.

TAKE A CHANCE:

- Use 1/8 teaspoon dried lavender instead of herbs de Provence.
- Cut the chicken into 1/4-inch cubes instead of shredding it.
- Add 3 teaspoons finely chopped black olives to the salad.
- Add some additional Garlic Mayonnaise before serving.

POACHING CHICKEN

Poaching chicken in a pot on the stove is really quite easy; but it's even easier when done in the microwave. Place the chicken breasts in a microwave bowl and add 1/2 cup water. Cover the bowl and cook on full power for 2 minutes. Turn the chicken and continue to cook in 1 minute segments until it is cooked through.

Chapter 4

Soups
With an Attitude

Coming home on a cold wintry day to a house that is warmed by the rich smell of simmering soup is one of life's simple but rewarding pleasures. In this chapter, you'll discover how garlic and onions enliven the flavor and enrich the appeal of soups from around the country and the world. Be sure to try such heartwarming creations as Scotland's traditional Cock-A-Leekie and our special version of Italy's famed Minestrone.

Chicken Broth Universal

Many cultures believe that a steaming mug of chicken broth or soup is a good remedy for just about any ailment, and we agree. Feel free to substitute this Chicken Broth with the Vegetable Broth in any of our recipes.

3-pound free-range chicken, skin removed

1 yellow or white onion, peeled and left whole

1 large carrot, quartered lengthwise

1 large celery rib with leaves, halved lengthwise

3 whole black peppercorns

YIELD: 6 SERVINGS   PREPARATION TIME: 1 HOUR

1. Place the chicken in a large pot with enough water to cover. Cover the pot and bring to a boil. Reduce the heat to medium-low and skim any foam from the water. Add the onion, carrot, celery, and peppercorns to the pot. Continue to simmer, uncovered, for 1 hour.

2. Remove the pot from the heat, cover, and allow to sit until the broth cools.

3. Using a large fork, transfer the chicken to a cutting board and slice or shred it as desired. Save for another use.

4. Using a slotted spoon, remove the vegetables and save them for another use.

5. Serve the broth immediately, or use it in another recipe.

TAKE A CHANCE:

• Use the white portion of 2 medium leeks or 4 sliced shallots instead of the onion.

Vegetable Broth United States

YIELD: 6 SERVINGS   PREPARATION TIME: 1 HOUR

1. Place all of the ingredients in a large pot and bring to a boil. Reduce the heat to medium-low, and simmer uncovered for 1 hour.

2. Using a slotted spoon, remove the vegetables and save them for another use.

3. Serve the broth immediately, or use in another recipe.

TAKE A CHANCE:

- Use the white portion of 2 medium leeks instead of the onion.

- For a fresh, clean taste, add ¼ cup lemon juice before serving.

Vegetable broth is used as the base for a variety of soups in many cultures. We use this broth as the basis for many of our soup recipes, as well as a flavorful ingredient in a number of other dishes.

8 cups water

2 teaspoons extra-virgin olive oil

1 yellow or white onion, peeled and left whole

2 cloves garlic, thinly sliced

2 carrots, quartered lengthwise

1 celery rib with leaves, halved lengthwise

2 potatoes, cut into ½-inch cubes

6 whole black peppercorns

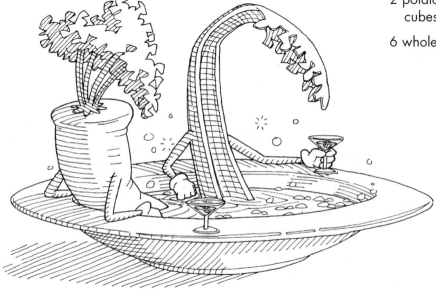

Garlic Broth France

The French consider garlic good for both the body and the soul. Slowly sip this garlicky broth from a mug, or use it as a base for a number of soups.

2 teaspoons extra-virgin olive oil

12 cloves garlic, thinly sliced

4 cups water

1 bay leaf

½ teaspoon freshly ground black pepper

YIELD: 4 SERVINGS   PREPARATION TIME: 25 MINUTES

1. Place the oil in a large saucepan over medium heat. Add the garlic and sauté for 2 minutes. Add the remaining ingredients and bring to a boil. Reduce the heat to medium, and simmer uncovered for 20 minutes.

2. Line a strainer with cheesecloth and strain the soup.

3. Return the broth to the pan and heat for 5 minutes before serving.

TAKE A CHANCE:

• Before serving, garnish with ½ cup sautéed leeks or scallions, or a dollop of Rouille (page 171).

• Use 2 fresh sage leaves instead of the bay leaf.

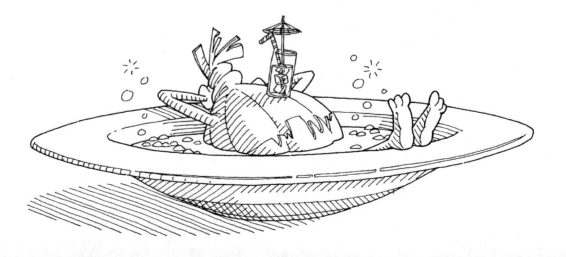

Onion Soup France

YIELD: 4 SERVINGS　　PREPARATION TIME: 1½ HOURS

1. Place ¼ cup of the broth and 2 tablespoons of margarine in a large pot over medium-low heat. Add the onions and black pepper and sauté about 30 minutes, or until the onions turn deep golden brown. Add the arrowroot and stir until well-mixed. Cook an additional 3 minutes.

2. Place the remaining broth in a saucepan and bring to a boil. Slowly add the hot broth to the onions, stirring constantly. Add the Worcestershire sauce. Simmer the soup, partially covered, for 30 minutes.

3. Melt the remaining margarine and spread it on both sides of the bread slices. Place the bread on a baking sheet and toast in a 350°F oven for 10 minutes. Place a piece of cheese on each slice of bread and sprinkle with Parmesan cheese. Continue to toast the bread for 5 minutes, or until the cheese has melted.

4. Place a piece of bread in the bottom of individual serving bowls, and ladle the soup on top. Serve immediately.

TAKE A CHANCE:

• Use Chicken Broth (page 58) instead of Vegetable Broth.

• Use an equal amount of onions and leeks instead of all onions.

• Add ⅛ teaspoon of cinnamon to the onions.

Slowly cooking the onions gives this classic French soup its rich, sweet taste.

5¼ cups Vegetable Broth (page 59)

4 tablespoons soy margarine

5 cups thinly sliced yellow or white onions

½ teaspoon freshly ground black pepper

1 tablespoon arrowroot

1 teaspoon Worcestershire sauce

4 slices French bread

4 slices Swiss cheese

2 teaspoons freshly grated Parmesan cheese

Onion & Bread Zuppa Italy

An Italian original, this delightful baked soup is flavored with red onions. When cooked, however, the onions lose their bright red color.

4 1/2 cups Chicken Broth (page 58)

6 red onions, thinly sliced

2 cups dry white wine

1/2 cinnamon stick

4 ounces stale Italian bread, broken into pieces

2 tablespoons freshly grated Romano cheese

YIELD: 6 SERVINGS   PREPARATION TIME: 1 1/2 HOURS

1. Heat 1/4 cup of the broth in a small saucepan over medium-low heat. Add the onions and sauté 5 minutes. Add the remaining broth, wine, and cinnamon, and bring to a boil.

2. Remove the pan from the stove and place the onion mixture in an ovenproof casserole dish.

3. Cover the casserole and place it in a 350°F oven for 1 hour. Remove the cover, mix in the bread, and continue to cook uncovered for another 20 minutes.

4. Remove the casserole dish from the oven, discard the cinnamon stick, and ladle the soup into a food processor. Pulse until the bread is broken up and the soup is smooth. Return the soup to a large saucepan and heat for 2 minutes.

5. Garnish with Romano cheese and serve hot or at room temperature.

TAKE A CHANCE:

• Use yellow or white onions instead of red ones.

• Use Vegetable Broth (page 59) instead of Chicken Broth.

Trivia Tidbit

Always wrap a cut onion before storing it in the refrigerator. This will keep the onion's pungent odor from invading other foods.

Onion Yogurt Soup United States

YIELD: 6 SERVINGS   PREPARATION TIME: 2 HOURS

1. Bring the broth to a boil in a large saucepan. Reduce the heat to medium-low and add the barley. Simmer uncovered for 30 minutes, or until the barley is tender. Transfer the soup to a large bowl and set aside.

2. In a small skillet, sauté the onion and garlic in the oil until the onion is soft, about 2 minutes. With a slotted spoon, remove the onion from the pan and add it to the broth. Cover the broth and let it cool to room temperature.

3. Combine the yogurt with the cooled broth. Cover and refrigerate until chilled, about 1 hour.

4. Before serving, stir the chilled soup well and garnish with mint.

TAKE A CHANCE:

- Use buckwheat instead of barley.
- Use chopped dill instead of mint.

A delicious summer soup. Bringing the broth to room temperature before mixing it with the yogurt will keep the soup from separating.

5 cups Vegetable Broth (page 59)

$1/2$ cup barley

1 yellow or white onion, coarsely chopped

2 cloves garlic, finely chopped

1 tablespoon canola oil

4 cups nonfat plain yogurt, at room temperature

$1/4$ cup finely chopped fresh mint

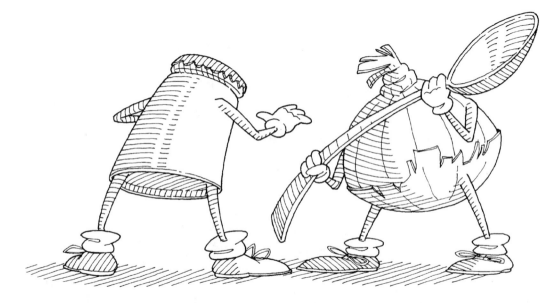

Garlic Soup Spain

This creamy-textured soup has a tangy garlic taste.

2 whole heads of garlic, finely chopped

4 cups Vegetable Broth (page 59)

$1/2$ cup egg substitute

2 tablespoons dry sherry (preferably Spanish)

2 tablespoons freshly grated Parmesan cheese

YIELD: 4 SERVINGS   PREPARATION TIME: 20 MINUTES

1. Place $1/4$ cup of the broth in a large saucepan over medium heat. Add the garlic and sauté for 2 minutes. Add the remaining broth and bring to a boil.

2. Reduce the heat to medium-low and simmer the broth for 10 minutes. Slowly add the egg and sherry to the broth and simmer for 5 minutes, or until the soup begins to thicken.

3. Garnish with Parmesan cheese and serve immediately.

TAKE A CHANCE:

• For a milder-tasting soup, don't chop the garlic cloves. Instead, drop the unpeeled cloves into boiling water for 2 minutes. Then peel the cloves and add them whole to the broth as it comes to a boil. Discard the cloves before serving the soup.

• Use Roasted Garlic (page 25) instead of raw.

• Use Chicken Broth (page 58) instead of Vegetable Broth.

Trivia Tidbit

The papery covering that encases the garlic head and the individual cloves is called a tunic.

Garlic Tomato Soup Cuba

1. Place the oil in a large saucepan over medium heat. Add the garlic and sauté for 2 minutes. Add the tomatoes and continue to cook for 10 minutes.

2. Reduce the heat to low and add the water, paprika, and black pepper. Cover and simmer for 5 minutes. Remove the lid and simmer another 10 minutes. Stir in the parsley.

3. Garnish the soup with Garlic Croutons and serve immediately.

TAKE A CHANCE:

• Just before serving, place the soup in a food processor and blend until smooth. Garnish with croutons and serve.

• Use Vegetable Broth (page 59) instead of water.

• Use chili powder instead of paprika.

Early Portuguese explorers brought garlic with them on their long sea voyages to Cuba. This recipe, which pairs garlic with a tomato-based soup, reflects the Portuguese influence on Cuban cuisine.

1 whole head garlic, coarsely chopped

1 tablespoon extra-virgin olive oil

8 medium tomatoes, peeled and coarsely chopped

6 cups water

1/2 teaspoon paprika

1/2 teaspoon freshly ground black pepper

1 tablespoon chopped fresh parsley

Garlic Croutons (page 158)

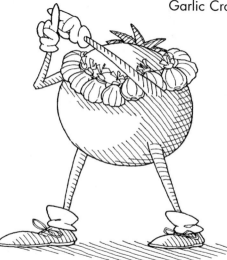

Vietnamese Soup Vietnam

In Vietnam, Buddhists use leeks in place of garlic and onions. Here, we've added leeks to bok choy (Chinese cabbage) for a satisfying soup.

4 ounces cellophane noodles*

5 cups Vegetable Broth (page 59)

2 tablespoons fish sauce (nuoc mam)*

2 cups coarsely chopped bok choy*

2 large leeks, white part only, thinly sliced

1 tablespoon canola oil or light sesame oil

2 tablespoons finely chopped cilantro

* Available in Asian markets, most gourmet shops, and some grocery stores.

YIELD: 4 SERVINGS   PREPARATION TIME: 30 MINUTES

1. Place the noodles in a medium bowl, cover with water, and soak for 10 minutes. Drain. Evenly divide the noodles and place in four soup bowls.

2. Combine the broth and fish sauce in a saucepan over medium heat. Just before the broth boils, remove the pan from the heat and set aside.

3. Place the oil in a large skillet over medium heat. Add the bok choy and leeks, and cook for 2 minutes, or until the bok choy wilts.

4. Place an equal amount of leeks and bok choy over the noodles in the soup bowls. Ladle the broth on top, garnish with cilantro, and serve immediately.

TAKE A CHANCE:

• Use rice noodles instead of cellophane noodles.

• Add 2 seeded and chopped Thai peppers or serrano chili peppers to the vegetables.

• Add $1/2$ cup diced tofu.

Basque Vegetable Soup Spain

YIELD: 6 SERVINGS PREPARATION TIME: 1 HOUR

1. Place all of the ingredients except the cabbage in a large pot. If necessary, add more water to completely cover the vegetables. Cover the pot and bring to a boil.

2. Reduce the heat to medium-low and simmer for 45 minutes. Add the cabbage and continue to cook another 10 minutes.

3. Serve immediately.

TAKE A CHANCE:

• Omit the turnip and add another potato.

Although the Basque region of Spain is close to the French border, this soup resembles Italian minestrone. It is a thick soup filled with onions, garlic, and leeks. We have omitted the salt pork and garlic sausage found in the traditional recipe.

6 cups water

1 cup cooked Great Northern white beans

1 yellow or white onion, thinly sliced

3 cloves garlic, thinly sliced

2 leeks, white part only, thinly sliced

2 carrots, cut into $1/2$-inch slices

2 potatoes, cut into $1/2$-inch cubes

1 sweet red pepper, cut into $1/2$-inch pieces

1 small turnip, cut into $1/2$-inch cubes

$1/2$ teaspoon thyme

$1/2$ teaspoon freshly ground black pepper

2 cups thinly sliced green cabbage

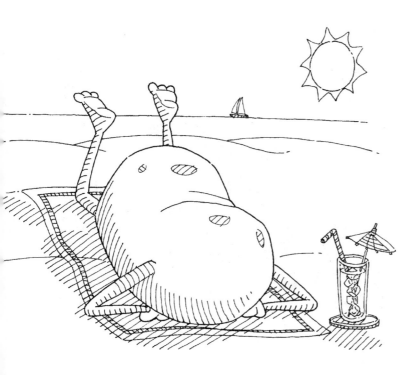

Minestrone Italy

This hearty soup will help chase away the winter blues. Take some along in a thermos to enjoy at a winter picnic or tailgate party.

6 cups Vegetable Broth (page 59)

1 yellow or white onion, coarsely chopped

1 carrot, cut into $1/2$-inch slices

2 potatoes, cut into $1/2$-inch cubes

2 celery ribs, sliced (leaves optional)

2 tomatoes, peeled, seeded, and coarsely chopped

2 zucchini, coarsely chopped

1 cup small pasta shells

2 tablespoons chopped Italian parsley

$1/4$ cup freshly grated Parmesan cheese

YIELD: 6 SERVINGS   PREPARATION TIME: 35 MINUTES

1. Place the broth in a large pot over medium heat. Add the onion, carrot, potatoes, celery, tomatoes, and zucchini, and simmer for 20 minutes. Add the pasta shells and cook until they are tender but not mushy.

2. Stir in the parsley, and serve immediately with Parmesan on the side.

TAKE A CHANCE:

- Use barley or rice instead of pasta.

- Omit 1 zucchini and add 1 chopped crookneck squash.

- Add 1 cup trimmed green beans, cut into 1–inch lengths.

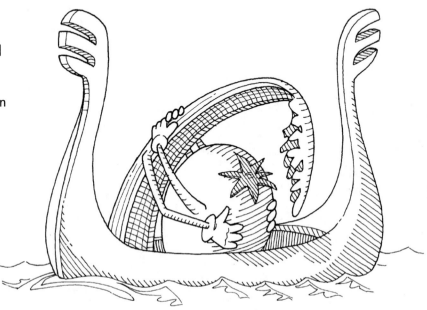

Vegetable Soup Pistou France

YIELD: 6 SERVINGS   PREPARATION TIME: 1 HOUR

1. To make the pistou, combine the garlic, basil, olive oil, and Parmesan in a food processor. Blend until smooth and set aside.

2. Bring the lentils and water to boil in a large pot. Reduce the heat to medium–low, cover, and simmer 30 minutes.

3. Add all of the remaining ingredients, except the pasta, and simmer 1 hour, or until the vegetables are tender. Add the pasta and cook uncovered for 10 minutes, or until the pasta is tender but not mushy.

4. Add the pistou, stir well, and serve immediately.

TAKE A CHANCE:

- Omit the cheese from the pistou and serve it on the side as a garnish instead.

Trivia Tidbit

Except for desserts, most recipes from Provence contain at least a small amount of some member of the allium family.

This classic soup from Provence is topped with pistou—a mixture of ground garlic, basil, and olive oil. Our version calls for lentils instead of the haricots and broad beans used in the traditional French recipe.

8 ounces dried lentils

6 cups water

1 yellow or white onion, finely chopped

2 leeks, white part only, thinly sliced

8 ounces green beans

1 potato, cut into cubes

2 zucchini, cut into cubes

2 tomatoes, seeded and coarsely chopped

3 whole fresh sage leaves

1/2 teaspoon freshly ground black pepper

8 ounces small pasta shells or vermicelli noodles

Pistou

4 cloves garlic

5 fresh basil leaves, torn in half

3 tablespoons extra-virgin olive oil

2 tablespoons freshly grated Parmesan cheese

Gazpacho Spain

There are hundreds of wonderful versions of this traditional cold soup like this one, with its mild red onion and lots of garlic. Replace the tomato juice with a tablespoon of olive oil and your soup becomes a salad.

3 large tomatoes, coarsely chopped

4 cloves garlic, finely chopped

1 red onion, coarsely chopped

1 cucumber, peeled, seeded, and coarsely chopped

1 small green pepper, coarsely chopped

1 jalapeño pepper, finely chopped

1 1/2 cups tomato juice

1/4 cup fresh lemon juice

10 drops hot sauce

1/4 teaspoon freshly ground black pepper

1/4 cup freshly chopped fresh cilantro

YIELD: 4 SERVINGS   PREPARATION TIME: 3 1/2 HOURS

1. Place all of the ingredients, except the cilantro, in a large bowl and stir well. Cover and refrigerate at least 3 hours.

2. Ladle the cold soup into bowls or mugs, garnish with cilantro, and serve.

TAKE A CHANCE:

• Use 3 chopped shallots instead of red onion

• Add 1/2 cup chopped zucchini or crookneck squash.

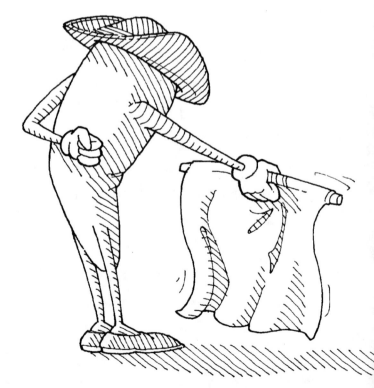

Black Bean Soup Central America

YIELD: 4 SERVINGS   PREPARATION TIME: 2½ HOURS

1. Place the beans in a large saucepan, cover with water, and bring to a boil. Reduce the heat and simmer until the beans are tender, about 1½ to 2 hours. Drain.

2. Place the oil in a large pot over medium heat. Add the onion and garlic, and sauté for 2 minutes. Add the jalapeños and chili powder, and sauté another minute. Add the cooked beans, broth, tomatoes, and black pepper. Simmer for 30 minutes.

3. Ladle the soup into bowls, garnish with a dollop of sour cream, and serve immediately.

TAKE A CHANCE:

• Use pinto beans instead of black beans.

• Use 2 cups tomato sauce instead of fresh tomatoes.

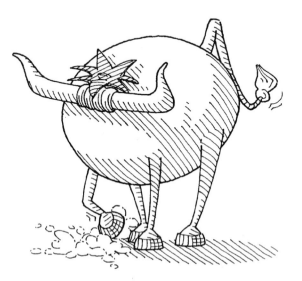

*B*lack beans are used exten-sively in the cuisine of Central America. Mixed with onions, garlic, and spices, this lively soup will warm you on a cold night.

1 cup dried black beans, rinsed

3 tablespoons canola oil

1 yellow or white onion, finely chopped

2 cloves garlic, finely chopped

3 jalapeño peppers, finely chopped

2 tablespoons chili powder

3 cups Vegetable Broth (page 59)

2 large tomatoes, seeded and coarsely chopped

¼ teaspoon freshly ground black pepper

4 tablespoons nonfat sour cream

Mushroom Barley Soup Russia

Filled with chewy barley and chunks of mushroom and onion, this soup goes a long way on a cold night. Pack some in a thermos for a warm pick-me-up on the slopes.

6 cups Vegetable Broth (page 59)

8 ounces mushrooms, coarsely sliced

1/2 cup pearl barley

1 yellow or white onion, coarsely chopped

2 carrots, thinly sliced

2 tablespoons chopped fresh dill, or 1 tablespoon dried

1/2 teaspoon freshly ground black pepper

YIELD: 6 SERVINGS   PREPARATION TIME: 2 HOURS

1. Bring the broth to a boil in a large pot. Reduce the heat to medium–low, add the mushrooms, and simmer for 30 minutes.

2. Add the remaining ingredients and continue to cook for 30 minutes, or until the barley is tender.

3. Serve immediately.

TAKE A CHANCE:

• Stir 1 tablespoon nonfat sour cream into each bowl of soup before serving.

• Add 1 diced potato.

Chicken Soup with Leeks & Tofu Japan

YIELD: 6 SERVINGS   PREPARATION TIME: 45 MINUTES

1. Bring the broth to a boil in a large pot. Reduce the heat to medium, add the chicken, and simmer for 15 minutes. Add the leeks, tofu, and shoyu, and continue to cook for 10 minutes. Stir in the lemon juice.

TAKE A CHANCE:

- Use 3 large, thinly sliced shallots instead of leeks.

- Use lime juice instead of lemon juice.

- For a vegetarian version, omit the chicken and use Vegetable Broth (page 59) instead of Chicken Broth.

- For added tartness, use more lemon juice.

Pieces of tofu and slices of leek give texture to this slightly tart chicken soup, which is traditionally sipped from a lacquered wooden bowl during the meal.

5 cups Chicken Broth (page 58)

2 skinless, boneless free-range chicken breasts, cut into $1/2$-inch pieces

2 large leeks, white part only, thinly sliced

4 ounces firm tofu, drained and cut into $1/4$-inch pieces

$1 1/2$ tablespoons shoyu or tamari soy sauce

3 tablespoons fresh lime juice

2 tablespoons finely chopped cilantro

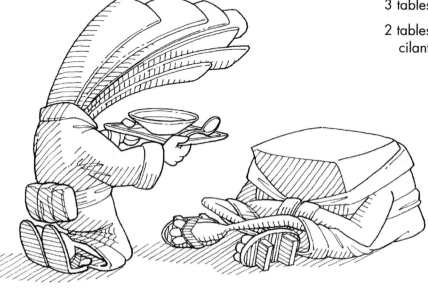

Cock-A-Leekie Scotland

Though not appreciated by everyone, the traditional prune placed at the bottom of each bowl adds a bit of sweetness to the mellow leeks and rich broth.

4 prunes, covered in cool water and soaked 8 hours or overnight

5 cups Chicken Broth (page 58)

4 leeks, white part only, thinly sliced

1 bay leaf

8 sprigs fresh parsley

4 whole black peppercorns

YIELD: 4 SERVINGS   PREPARATION TIME: 45 MINUTES

1. Drain the prunes and set aside.

2. Place $1/4$ cup of the broth in a large pot over medium heat. Add the leeks and sauté for 2 minutes. Add the bay leaf, parsley, peppercorns, and the remaining broth, and bring to a boil.

3. Reduce the temperature to medium, and simmer the soup uncovered for 30 minutes. Add the prunes and continue to cook for 10 minutes.

4. Remove the parsley and bay leaf from the pot and discard.

5. Place a prune in the bottom of each bowl and ladle the soup on top.

TAKE A CHANCE:

- Use $1/2$ cup raisins instead of prunes.

- Omit the prunes altogether.

- Add 1 cup of chopped chicken to the broth before serving.

Potato Leek Soup Poland

YIELD: 6 SERVINGS PREPARATION TIME: 1 HOUR

1. Melt the margarine in a small saucepan over medium-low heat. Add the leeks and sauté for 20 minutes.

2. Bring the broth to a boil in a large pot. Reduce the heat to medium-low, add the potatoes, and cook uncovered for 20 minutes. Add the sautéed leeks, black pepper, and caraway seeds. Continue to cook for 5 minutes.

3. Serve immediately.

TAKE A CHANCE:

- Add ¼ cup diced carrots to the pot along with the potatoes.

- Omit the caraway seeds and garnish with 2 tablespoons chopped fresh parsley or dill.

- Omit the caraway seeds and garnish with Garlic Croutons (page 158).

This soup, which concentrates on the goodness of leeks and potatoes, has a small surprise—caraway seeds.

4 leeks, white part only, thinly sliced

2 tablespoons soy margarine

4 cups Chicken Broth (page 58)

4 potatoes, cut into ¼-inch cubes

½ teaspoon freshly ground black pepper

1 tablespoon caraway seeds

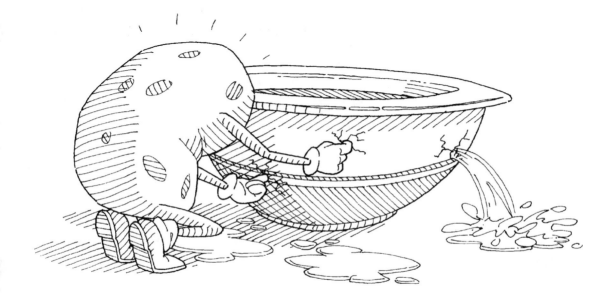

Bacon Leek Soup Germany

This creamy soup with bits of bacon has a flavorful secret ingredient—a dash of nutmeg.

3 strips soy bacon, cooked, drained, and crumbled

3 leeks, white part only, thinly sliced

4$^1/2$ cups Vegetable Broth (page 59)

2 tablespoons arrowroot

3 tablespoons skim milk

$^1/2$ teaspoon freshly ground black pepper

$^1/8$ teaspoon nutmeg

1 egg yolk

2 tablespoons cold water

YIELD: 6 SERVINGS   PREPARATION TIME: 30 MINUTES

1. Place $^1/2$ cup of the broth in a large pot over medium heat. Add the leeks and sauté for 5 minutes. Add the bacon and 1 tablespoon of the arrowroot, and cook for 2 minutes. Slowly add the remaining broth while stirring constantly. Simmer uncovered for 10 minutes.

2. In a small bowl, blend the milk and the remaining arrowroot. Add 2 tablespoons of the warm broth to the bowl, mix well, then slowly stir into the pot. Bring the soup to a boil, reduce the heat to medium-low, and add the pepper and nutmeg.

3. In a small bowl, lightly beat together the egg yolk and water. Slowly add this mixture to the soup while stirring constantly.

4. Serve immediately.

TAKE A CHANCE:

• Use Chicken Broth (page 58) instead of Vegetable Broth.

• Omit the bacon.

• Instead of adding the nutmeg to the soup, sprinkle it on top of the individual servings.

Chunky Leek & Vegetable Soup Bulgaria

YIELD: 6 SERVINGS PREPARATION TIME: 1 HOUR

1. Place $1/2$ cup of the broth in a large pot over medium heat. Add the leeks, and sauté 2 minutes. Add the carrot and continue to sauté for 5 minutes. Add the remaining broth, potatoes, and black pepper, and bring to a boil.

2. Reduce the heat to medium–low, cover, and simmer for 20 minutes. Add the zucchini and continue to simmer for 20 minutes, or until the vegetables are cooked.

3. Garnish with parsley and serve immediately.

TAKE A CHANCE:

• Use crookneck squash instead of zucchini.

• Use fresh dill instead of parsley.

Leeks make this chunky soup a real crowd pleaser.

6$1/2$ cups Vegetable Broth (page 59)

5 leeks, white part only, cut lengthwise then crosswise into $1/4$-inch pieces

1 carrot, cut into $1/4$-inch slices

2 potatoes, cut into $1/2$-inch cubes

$1/2$ teaspoon freshly ground black pepper

2 zucchini, cut lengthwise then crosswise into $1/2$-inch pieces

2 tablespoons finely chopped fresh parsley

Creamy Leek & Potato Soup Wales

*L*eeks are one of very few root vegetables that are indigenous to Wales. Here they are paired with potatoes and onion in a satisfying soup.

5 cups Vegetable Broth (page 59)

3 leeks, white part only, thinly sliced

4 potatoes, cut into $\frac{1}{2}$-inch cubes

1 yellow or white onion, thinly sliced

$\frac{1}{2}$ cup skim milk

$\frac{1}{4}$ teaspoon freshly ground black pepper

YIELD: 6 SERVINGS   PREPARATION TIME: 1 HOUR

1. Bring the broth to a boil in a large saucepan, then reduce the heat to medium–low. Add the leeks, potatoes, and onion, and simmer covered for 25 to 30 minutes, or until the potatoes are cooked.

2. To the pot, add the milk and black pepper and stir well. Cover and simmer for 5 minutes, or until the broth is heated.

3. Serve immediately.

TAKE A CHANCE:

• Use Chicken Broth (page 58) instead of Vegetable Broth.

• Omit the milk.

Trivia Tidbit

Leeks hold an honored place in Welsh history. In the sixth century, on the suggestion of David, the patron saint of Wales, Welsh warriors wore leeks tucked into their caps to distinguish themselves from the invading Saxon army.

Fish Soup Norway

YIELD: 6 SERVINGS   PREPARATION TIME: 30 MINUTES

1. Melt the margarine in a large skillet over low heat, add the leeks, and sauté for 2 minutes. Add the celery and sauté another minute. Add the potatoes and continue sautéing 2 more minutes. Increase the heat to medium, add the water, and continue cooking for 10 minutes. The vegetables should be slightly hard.

2. Add the fish, dill, and black pepper, and continue to cook for 5 minutes, or until the vegetables are tender and the fish is cooked.

3. Garnish with scallions and serve immediately.

TAKE A CHANCE:

- Add the scallions to the soup and garnish with the dill.
- Sauté 1/2 cup diced green pepper along with the celery.

Tiny morsels of fish are enhanced by leeks and scallions in this Norwegian fish soup. If you find the fresh dill hard to chop, snip it directly into the soup with a pair of clean scissors.

1 tablespoon soy margarine

2 leeks, white part only, thinly sliced

1 celery rib, coarsely diced

3 potatoes, cut into 1/2-inch cubes

5 cups water

1 pound white fish, such as cod or flounder, cut into 1-inch pieces

1 teaspoon finely chopped fresh dill, or 1/2 teaspoon dried

1/2 teaspoon freshly ground black pepper

2 scallions, finely chopped

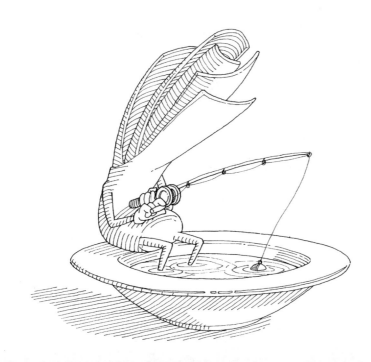

Down South Gumbo United States

Gumbo is served throughout the Louisiana bayou. There are almost as many gumbo recipes as there are people living in that state. This is our official version of this favorite Southern dish. Serve it with steaming hot rice on the side.

8 1/4 cups Chicken Broth (page 58)

3-pound free-range chicken, skinned and cut into 8 pieces

3 tablespoons canola oil

3 tablespoons unbleached flour

1 cup finely chopped scallions

3 cloves garlic, finely chopped

2 celery ribs, finely chopped

1 green bell pepper, finely chopped

2 teaspoons cayenne pepper

1/2 teaspoon freshly ground black pepper

1 teaspoon filé powder*

1/4 cup finely chopped fresh parsley

* A traditional thickening agent used in Creole gumbos, filé (powdered sassafras leaves) is available in gourmet shops and some grocery stores.

YIELD: 10 SERVINGS   PREPARATION TIME: 1 HOUR

1. Place 1/4 cup of broth in a large pot over medium heat. Add the chicken and sauté until golden brown. Transfer the chicken to a dish that is lined with paper toweling. Cover and set aside to cool.

2. Add the oil and flour to the pot and stir with a spoon until the mixture turns nutty brown, about 5 minutes. Add the scallions, garlic, celery, and green pepper, and cook over medium-low heat for 2 minutes.

3. Very slowly, pour the remaining broth into the pot, stirring constantly to avoid lumps. Bring the broth to a boil, then reduce the heat to low. Add the cayenne and black pepper, mix well, and simmer uncovered for 25 minutes.

4. Remove the bones from the chicken and shred the meat. Add the chicken to the gumbo and continue to simmer for 15 minutes. Remove the pot from the heat and stir in the filé powder.

5. Ladle the gumbo into bowls, garnish with parsley, and serve immediately.

TAKE A CHANCE:

• Add 1 cup chopped okra to the pot along with the other vegetables.

• Use 1 tablespoon hot sauce instead of cayenne pepper.

Chapter 5

Vegetarian Main Meals
Nothing Dull on This Plate

Sometimes vegetarian fare has a reputation for being dull, especially to those who are tired of those three-bean salads and tofu burgers. If you are one who feels this way, simply try a few of the recipes in this chapter to see how just easy it is to put a little passion in a vegetarian meal. The secret? Just keep those fresh onions, leeks, and garlic on hand. They will enliven any dish, and your tastebuds will thank you for it.

Wrapped Tofu Greece

*O*riginally made with lamb by bandits hiding out in the Greek mountains, this vegetarian version loses none of the flavor. It's always fun to watch as people peek to see what's inside the pouches.

Marinade

4 cloves garlic, finely chopped

¼ cup fresh lemon juice

1 teaspoon dried oregano

½ teaspoon dried basil

Pouches

1 pound firm tofu, drained and cut lengthwise into four 1-inch slices

1 tomato, thinly sliced

4 ounces feta cheese, crumbled

1 yellow or white onion, sliced into thin rings

½ teaspoon dried oregano

½ teaspoon freshly ground black pepper

1 tablespoon finely chopped parsley

4 tablespoons fresh lemon juice

1. Combine the marinade ingredients in a small bowl and let sit for 5 minutes.

2. Place the tofu in a large bowl and pour the marinade on top. Cover and refrigerate for 1 hour, turning the tofu at least once.

3. Arrange four 12-x-12-inch sheets of aluminum foil on the counter. Place a piece of tofu on the middle of each sheet, and top with equal amounts of tomato, feta cheese, and onion rings. Sprinkle each with equal amounts of oregano, black pepper, and parsley.

4. Bring up the sides of the foil and carefully pour a tablespoon of lemon juice over the ingredients in each packet.

5. Tightly crimp together the foil edges to form packets. Place on a baking sheet and bake in a preheated 350°F oven for 20 minutes, or until the cheese is melted and the tofu is heated through.

6. Serve immediately with Spicy Steamed Vegetables (page 144).

TAKE A CHANCE:

• Add 2 tablespoons dry white wine to the marinade.

• Use chicken breasts or lamb instead of tofu.

Stuffed Tofu Southeast Asia

1. To make the filling, place the broth in a large skillet over medium heat. Add the onion, shallots, and garlic, and sauté for 1 minute. Add the soy sauce, ginger, and black pepper, and sauté another minute.

2. Using a sharp knife, carefully cut a pocket into the side of the tofu. Remove enough tofu to leave a $1/2$-inch-thick shell. Stuff the pocket with the filling, and place it in a $1^1/2$-quart casserole dish that has been lightly coated with cooking spray. Set aside.

3. Place the sesame seeds in a small ungreased skillet and toast until golden brown. Remove the skillet from the heat and cool for 2 minutes. Add the sesame oil, lemon juice, and scallions to the skillet, and mix well with the sesame seeds. Return the skillet to the stove and sauté the sesame mixture over medium heat for 2 minutes.

4. Pour the sesame mixture over the tofu and bake in a 350°F for 20 minutes, or until the tofu is warmed through.

5. Place the stuffed tofu on a serving platter and pour the cooking juices on top. Serve with Grilled Vegetable Kebabs (page 148).

TAKE A CHANCE:

• Add $1/4$ cup cooked chicken or chopped walnuts to the filling.

• Instead of onion filling, stuff the tofu with Gremolata (page 172).

• Instead of stuffing the tofu, cut it into $1/2$-inch pieces and sauté it with the onions. Add the sesame oil, lemon juice, and scallions, and continue sautéing. Garnish with sesame seeds and serve.

• Top with Onion Sauce (page 163) or Onion Gravy (page 164) instead of the cooking juices.

Tofu is popular among many cultures of Southeast Asia. In this recipe, the tofu absorbs the onion and garlic flavor for a heavenly taste.

1 pound firm tofu, drained

2 tablespoons sesame seeds

2 tablespoons sesame oil

3 tablespoons fresh lemon juice

2 scallions, coarsely chopped

Filling

3 tablespoons Vegetable Broth (page 59)

1 sweet onion, such as Vidalia, Walla Walla, or Spanish, coarsely chopped

2 shallots, coarsely chopped

3 cloves garlic, coarsely chopped

2 tablespoons shoyu or tamari soy sauce

$1/2$ teaspoon freshly grated ginger

$1/4$ teaspoon freshly ground black pepper

Sauerbraten Germany

Tofu's porous texture absorbs the piquant sauerbraten marinade. The garnish gives this dish a spark of color.

1½ pounds firm tofu, drained and cut into 1-inch cubes

2 tablespoons safflower oil

1 cup coarsely chopped yellow or white onions

1 tablespoon arrowroot

1 cup Vegetable Broth (page 59)

1 tablespoon date sugar

¼ cup grated carrot

3 tablespoons finely chopped fresh parsley

Marinade

1 cup water

¼ cup lemon juice

2 tablespoons white vinegar

1 cup coarsely chopped yellow or white onions

4 cloves garlic, finely chopped

1 celery rib, thinly sliced

1 carrot, thinly sliced

1 tablespoon grated ginger

3 whole cloves, or ¼ teaspoon ground

3 whole black peppercorns

YIELD: 4 SERVINGS   PREPARATION TIME: 2 DAYS

1. Bring the marinade ingredients to a boil in a saucepan.

2. Place the tofu in a large bowl, add the marinade, and mix well. Cover and refrigerate for 1½ days, stirring the tofu at least 3 times. Remove the marinated tofu to a plate and set aside. With a slotted spoon, remove and discard the vegetables from the marinade. Reserve the marinade.

3. Place the oil in a large skillet over medium heat. Add the onion and sauté until brown, about 10 minutes. Add the arrowroot and stir constantly for 1 minute. Gradually add the broth, the reserved marinade, and the sugar. Stirring constantly, bring the mixture to a boil. Reduce the heat to medium-low and add the tofu. Cover and simmer for 20 minutes, or until the sauce thickens slightly.

4. Spoon over plain rice or noodles. Garnish with carrots and parsley. Serve with Braised Red Cabbage (page 138).

TAKE A CHANCE:

- Use half onions and half leeks instead of all onions.

- Garnish with Gremolata (page 172) instead of carrots and parsley.

- Reduce the Vegetable Broth amount to ½ cup and add ½ cup dry red wine.

- For additional color, add ½ cup diced red bell pepper to the tofu as it simmers.

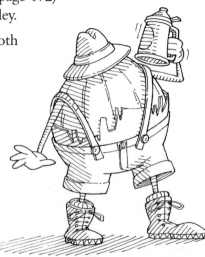

Fried Rice China

*T*his basic recipe for fried rice is filled with chopped scallions. Feel free to add cooked chicken or shrimp, or your favorite vegetables.

1. Place 1 tablespoon of the oil in a wok or skillet over medium heat. Slowly add the egg mixture, stirring constantly until the egg is cooked dry and broken into pieces. Remove the eggs to a heated dish and set aside.

2. Heat the remaining oil over medium-high heat for 1 minute. Add the rice and scallions, and stir-fry for 5 minutes. Stir in the broth, soy sauce, and black pepper, and continue to cook for 2 minutes. Add the cooked eggs and sesame oil and stir well.

3. Place the cooked rice in a serving bowl and enjoy immediately.

TAKE A CHANCE:

• Add $^1/_4$ cup each of peas and diced carrots.

• Add $^1/_2$ cup snow peas.

$^1/_2$ cup egg substitute, or 2 beaten eggs

3 tablespoons canola oil

4 cups cooked rice (cold)

$^1/_2$ cup finely chopped scallions

3 tablespoons Vegetable Broth (page 59)

2 tablespoons shoyu or tamari soy sauce

$^1/_2$ teaspoon freshly ground black pepper

1 teaspoon light sesame oil

Garlic Vegetable Pizza Italy

*F*resh vegetables dot this incredible pizza, which is covered with mounds of melted cheese and lots of garlic.

Crust

1 package dry active yeast

1 tablespoon honey

1 cup lukewarm water

1 cup whole wheat pastry flour

2 tablespoons canola oil

2 cups unbleached flour

1 tablespoon cornmeal

Marinade

8 cloves garlic, crushed

2 teaspoons extra-virgin olive oil

2 teaspoons fresh lemon juice

2 teaspoons finely chopped fresh oregano, or 1 teaspoon dried

Topping

1/4 cup finely chopped yellow or white onions

1/2 cup broccoli florets, cut in half

1/2 cup fresh spinach leaves

2 tomatoes, thinly sliced

YIELD: 4 INDIVIDUAL OR 2 MEDIUM-SIZED PIZZAS
PREPARATION TIME: 1 1/2 HOURS

1. To prepare the crust, dissolve the yeast and honey in the water in a large bowl. Allow to sit for 5 minutes.

2. Stir the pastry flour and oil into the yeast mixture. Add the unbleached flour 1/2 cup at a time, mixing until a soft dough forms. Turn the dough onto a lightly floured board and knead until smooth and elastic. If the dough is sticky, add more flour, a little at a time.

3. Form the dough into a ball and place it in a large bowl that is coated with oil or a nonstick spray. Turn the dough over once to coat both sides with the oil. Cover the bowl with wax paper and a clean towel, and set in a warm place for 45 minutes, or until the dough doubles in size.

4. While the dough is rising, combine the marinade ingredients together in a large bowl. Add the onions, broccoli, spinach, tomatoes, and zucchini to the bowl, stir well, and marinate for 30 minutes.

5. When the dough has doubled, punch it down and remove it from the bowl. Cut the dough in half for 2 medium-sized pizzas or in quarters for 4 individual pies.

6. Sprinkle the board with cornmeal and place a ball of dough on top. Flatten the dough with the heel of your hand, then carefully stretch it to the desired size. Place the dough on a pizza pan or baking sheet and, using your fingertips, form a 1/2-inch rim around the crust. Repeat with the other portions of dough.

7. Top the dough with the marinated vegetables, and the mozzarella and Parmesan cheeses. Place on the lowest rack in a preheated 500°F oven, and bake until the cheese is melted and the crust is brown and crisp, about 10 to 15 minutes.

8. Remove the pizza from the oven and let it stand for 5 minutes before cutting and serving.

TAKE A CHANCE:

• Use elephant garlic instead of regular garlic.

• Add a clove or two of crushed garlic to the dough.

• Instead of marinating the onions, sauté them in a tablespoon of olive oil. When cooled, add them to the pizza along with the remaining vegetables.

• Roast 3 heads of garlic (page 25). Crush the cloves, mix them with the cheese and vegetables, and spread the mixture over the dough. Cook according to the instructions in step 7.

¼ cup thinly sliced zucchini

1 cup freshly grated mozzarella cheese

2 teaspoons freshly grated Parmesan cheese

FREEZING PIZZA DOUGH

Pizza dough can be made ahead of time and stored in the freezer. Once the formed dough has risen, punch it down. Coat the dough with cornmeal, wrap it securely in plastic, and place it in the freezer where it will keep for several weeks. When you are ready to use the dough, defrost it at room temperature for 2 to 4 hours or in the refrigerator overnight.

Navajo Tacos American Southwest

*I*nspired by the tacos made on
Arizona's Navajo reservations,
these savory open-faced tacos are
very satisfying. Instead of wrap-
ping the filling in traditional taco
shells, we pile it on crisp pizza
crusts.

Crust

1 package active dry yeast

1 tablespoon honey

1 cup lukewarm water

3 cups whole wheat pastry
   flour

2 tablespoons canola oil

Filling

2 teaspoons safflower oil

2 yellow or white onions,
   finely chopped

3 cloves garlic, finely chopped

$1/2$ teaspoon chili powder

3 cups cooked pinto beans

Toppings

1 cup shredded lettuce

1 cup coarsely chopped
   tomatoes

1 cup grated cheddar cheese

YIELD: 4 MEDIUM-SIZED TACOS
PREPARATION TIME: $1^3/4$ HOURS

1. To prepare the crust, dissolve the yeast and honey in the water
   in a large bowl. Allow to sit for 5 minutes.

2. Stir the oil into the yeast mixture. Add the unbleached flour
   $1/2$ cup at a time, mixing until a soft dough forms. Turn the
   dough onto a lightly floured work surface and knead until
   smooth and elastic. If the dough is sticky, add more flour, a little at a time.

3. Form the dough into a ball and place it in a large bowl that is
   coated with oil or a nonstick spray. Turn dough over once to
   coat both sides with the oil. Cover the bowl with wax paper
   and a clean towel, and set in a warm place for 45 minutes, or
   until the dough doubles in size.

4. When the dough has doubled, punch it down and remove it
   from the bowl. Cut the dough into quarters.

5. Sprinkle the work surface with cornmeal and place a piece of
   dough on top. Flatten the dough with the heel of your hand,
   then carefully stretch it to the desired size. Place the flattened
   dough on a pizza pan or baking sheet and, using your fingertips, form a $1/2$-inch rim around the crust. Repeat with the
   other portions of dough.

6. Place the baking sheet on the lowest rack in a preheated 500°F
   oven and bake the crusts for 10 minutes or until they are
   brown. Remove from the oven and let stand for 5 minutes.

7. While the crusts are baking, prepare the filling. Place the oil in
   a large skillet over medium heat. Add the onions and garlic,
   and sauté for 5 minutes. Add the chili powder and sauté
   another minute. Add the pinto beans and continue to cook
   until they are heated through.

8. Evenly divide the bean filling on the pizza shells. Top with lettuce, tomatoes, and cheese. Serve immediately.

TAKE A CHANCE:

• Serve on whole wheat tortillas or Indian Fry Bread (page 189).

• Add 2 seeded, chopped jalapeño peppers to the filling mixture.

• Use red kidney beans instead of pinto beans.

• Add $1/2$ cup of your favorite meat substitute to the filling.

CHILI PEPPERS

The small but powerful chili pepper, which comes in over a hundred varieties, adds distinct character—and varying degrees of heat—to any dish. Living in the western part of the United States, we are lucky to have access to an outrageous variety of these potent gems. On our last cross-country trip, we were happy to discover that a great number of chili peppers are becoming more readily available throughout the country.

Here's a brief description of the most frequently used chili peppers called for in our recipes.

Habeñero. This lantern-shaped chili, also known as a "Scotch Bonnet," ranges in color from light green and yellow to orange and bright red. Considered one of the hottest varieties, habañeros, rate a 10 on the heat scale.

Jalapeño. One of the best-known and most readily available chili peppers, jalapeños are usually green or red, and rate a 5 on the heat scale.

Serrano. This small, thin-skinned pepper comes in a range of colors like the habañero, and scores a 7 on the heat scale.

Thai. It's hard to imagine Thai food without chili peppers, but it wasn't until the New World was discovered that they made their way to Thailand (Siam). Developed in the early sixteenth century, Thai peppers are two or three inches long and rate an 8 on the heat scale.

To cut down on the heat of a chili pepper, simply remove its seeds. And be careful—when handling any chili peppers, always wear gloves and be very careful not to touch your eyes. Hot pepper juice can have a devastating, long-lasting effect.

Bean Curd Kung Pao China

The Chinese call it bean curd, while the Japanese name may be more familiar to you—tofu. This is a tasty dish regardless of what you call the main ingredient.

1 pound bean curd, drained and cut into 1-inch pieces

3 tablespoons canola or light sesame oil

5 dried Szechuan chili peppers*

1/2 cup dry-roasted peanuts

6 Szechuan peppercorns,* or whole black peppercorns

1 yellow or white onion, finely chopped

2 cloves garlic, minced

1 teaspoon freshly grated ginger

3 scallions, trimmed and diagonally cut into 1 1/2-inch pieces

Marinade

2 tablespoons dry sherry

2 tablespoons shoyu or tamari soy sauce

2 tablespoons arrowroot

* Available in Asian markets, gourmet shops, and some grocery stores.

YIELD: 4 SERVINGS   PREPARATION TIME: 1 HOUR

1. Place the bean curd in a large bowl. Mix the marinade ingredients together and pour it over the bean curd. Stir well, cover, and marinate at room temperature for 30 minutes.

2. Place 1 tablespoon of the oil in a wok or large skillet over medium heat. Add the peppers, peanuts, and peppercorns, and sauté for 2 minutes. Remove the ingredients to a plate.

3. Add the remaining oil to the wok and increase the heat to medium-high. Add the onion, garlic, and ginger, and sauté for 1 minute. Add the bean curd and marinade, and stir-fry for 5 minutes. Return the sautéed pepper–peanut mixture to the wok. Add the scallions and continue to cook for 5 minutes, or until the sauce starts to thicken.

4. Serve immediately with Fried Rice (page 85).

TAKE A CHANCE:

- Add 1/4 cup mushrooms and 1/4 cup snow peas to the wok along with the bean curd.

- Use 3 seeded and minced serrano or Thai chili peppers instead of the Szechuan chili peppers.

- Use Scallion Oil (recipe found under Scallion Sauce on page 165) instead of canola oil.

- Use cubed chicken breasts instead of the tofu.

Trivia Tidbit

The use of garlic and scallions is characteristic of the cooking style of Northern China.

Shepherd's Pie England

This recipe will feed a crowd, or at least a very hungry family.

YIELD: 6 SERVINGS   PREPARATION TIME: 1½ HOURS

1. Place $^1/_4$ cup of the broth in a large skillet over medium heat. Add the onions and garlic, and sauté for 5 minutes. Add the soybeans and continue to cook for 10 minutes.

2. To the skillet, add the tomato paste, another $^1/_2$ cup of broth, and the arrowroot, stirring until the arrowroot is completely dissolved. Add the wine, sage, and black pepper, mix well, and cook uncovered for 20 minutes.

3. While the soybean mixture is cooking, boil the potatoes until they are fork tender. Drain the potatoes and place them in a food processor along with the remaining broth. Pulse until smooth, adding additional broth if necessary.

4. Coat a 2-quart casserole with nonstick cooking spray. Spoon the soybean mixture into the dish and spread it evenly on the bottom. Spread the mashed potatoes over the mixture. Bake in a preheated 350°F oven for 35 minutes, then place it under the broiler for 2 to 3 minutes to brown the top.

5. Garnish with chives and serve with Crunchy Cucumber Salad (page 155) or Pickled Onions (page 48).

TAKE A CHANCE:

- Add $^1/_4$ cup each corn and diced red bell pepper to the soybean mixture.

- Omit the chives. Sprinkle 1 tablespoon Parmesan cheese over the potatoes before baking.

- Use Garlic Mashed Potatoes (page 127).

1 $^1/_4$ cups Vegetable Broth (page 59)

2 yellow or white onions, finely chopped

2 cloves garlic, finely chopped

3 cups cooked soybeans, or your favorite veggie burger mix

6 ounces tomato paste

1 tablespoon arrowroot

1 cup dry white wine

$^1/_2$ teaspoon dried sage

$^1/_4$ teaspoon freshly ground black pepper

3 large russet potatoes, quartered

2 teaspoon chopped chives

Stuffed Burgers with Sweet Onion United States

There's nothing quite like the taste of a barbecued burger topped with a thick, crunchy slice of grilled sweet onion.

Burger Mixture

1¹/₂ pounds of your favorite soy- or veggie-burger mix

3 tablespoons toasted bread crumbs

3 cloves garlic, crushed

¹/₂ teaspoon Worcestershire sauce

¹/₂ teaspoon ground sage

¹/₂ teaspoon ground thyme

¹/₄ teaspoon freshly ground black pepper

1 egg white

Filling

¹/₄ cup thinly sliced mushrooms

4 jalapeño peppers, seeded and finely chopped

2 ounces feta cheese, crumbled

Topping

1 sweet onion such, as Vidalia, cut into ¹/₂-inch slices

YIELD: 4 BURGERS   PREPARATION TIME: 45 MINUTES

1. Combine the burger mixture ingredients in a large bowl and mix well. Shape into 8 thin patties about 4 inches in diameter.

2. Top 4 of the patties with equal amounts of mushrooms, jalapeño peppers, and cheese, keeping this filling to within 1 inch of the edges. Place the remaining patties on top. Seal the edges by pinching the two patties together. Make sure none of the filling falls out.

3. Place the burgers on a hot barbecue grill and cook for 5 to 10 minutes on each side, or until they are cooked through.

4. While the burgers are cooking, place the onion slices on the grill and cook them 1 to 2 minutes on each side.

5. Top the burgers with the grilled onions and serve immediately with Tomato Salad (page 47).

TAKE A CHANCE:

• Instead of grilling the onion, cut it into very thin slices and sauté in a skillet with 2 tablespoons of canola oil. Sauté for 10 to 15 minutes, or until the slices are deep brown.

• Serve the burgers with Backyard Barbecue Sauce (page 162).

• Turn your burgers into mini loaves. Instead of grilling, bake them in a 350°F oven for 25 minutes, or until they are cooked through. Serve with Onion Gravy (page 164).

• Use a sliced red onion instead of a sweet onion.

Vegetable Quesadillas Mexico

YIELD: 4 TORTILLAS   PREPARATION TIME: 20 MINUTES

1. Place the oil in a small skillet over medium heat. Add the mushrooms and sauté for 1 minute. Add the zucchini and nopales, and sauté for another minute.

2. Place the tortillas on a clean, flat surface. Sprinkle some of the cheese over half of each tortilla, to within $1/2$-inch of the edge. Evenly layer all of the remaining ingredients, except for the Salsa Cruda, on the cheese, then top with the remaining cheese.

3. Fold the tortillas in half and place on a baking sheet. Bake in a 350°F oven for 5 minutes, or until the cheese begins to melt.

4. Serve immediately with Salsa Cruda.

TAKE A CHANCE:

• Sauté 1 finely minced garlic clove along with the other vegetables.

• Use crookneck squash instead of zucchini.

• Sauté $1/2$ cup chopped spinach with the other vegetables.

• Use mozzarella cheese instead of Monterey Jack.

• Use 3 or 4 seeded and finely minced serranos or poblano chilies instead of nopales.

Quesadillas, which can serve as appetizers or light meals, are very easy to make. We use vegetables in this recipe, but feel free to add your favorite taco or burrito filling for a more substantial meal.

4 large flour tortillas

1 teaspoon safflower oil

$1/2$ cup thinly sliced mushrooms

$1/2$ cup zucchini, cut into matchstick-sized pieces

$1/2$ cup peeled and boiled nopales (cactus paddles)*

$1/2$ cup shredded Monterey Jack cheese

$1/4$ cup finely chopped red onion

2 jalapeño peppers, seeded and finely chopped

2 tablespoons finely chopped cilantro

1 cup Salsa Cruda (page 22)

*Available fresh or bottled in gourmet and specialty stores. If using the bottled variety, rinse and drain before using.

Hearty Vegetable Ragout France

*B*ased on a classic French recipe for ratatouille, this dish includes all of our favorite alliums.

1/4 cup Vegetable Broth (page 59)

1 yellow or white onion, finely chopped

2 cloves garlic, thinly sliced

4 shallots, thinly sliced

2 large leeks, white part only, thinly sliced

2 zucchini, cut into 1/2-inch pieces

1 crookneck squash, cut into 1/2-inch slices

8 ounces large white mushrooms, quartered

1 medium eggplant, peeled and cut into 1/2-inch cubes

1 cup tomato sauce

1/4 teaspoon dried marjoram

2 tablespoons finely chopped fresh chives

YIELD: 4 SERVINGS   PREPARATION TIME: 1 HOUR

1. Place the broth in a large skillet over medium heat. Add the onion, garlic, and shallots, and sauté for 2 minutes. Add the leeks and sauté another minute. Add the zucchini, squash, mushrooms, and eggplant, and continue to sauté for 2 minutes.

2. Reduce the heat to low, add the tomato sauce and marjoram, and mix well. Cover and simmer for 30 minutes, stirring occasionally and adding more water or broth if the vegetables seem dry.

3. Transfer the vegetables to a large bowl and mix well. Garnish with the chives and serve immediately with Pissaladiere (page 187).

TAKE A CHANCE:

• Add 2 sliced green bell peppers to the vegetables.

• For a spicier taste, add 1 teaspoon dried red pepper flakes to the shallots and garlic.

Trivia Tidbit

Reconstitute dried chives by immersing them in fresh lemon juice.

Vegetable Curry Pakistan

Yield: 4 Servings   Preparation Time: 30 Minutes

1. Place the rice in a large bowl and cover with cold water. Rub the grains with your fingers, then drain. Repeat this process 4 more times, then let the rice drain.

2. Place $1/4$ cup of the broth in a large skillet over medium heat. Add the garlic, cumin, coriander, turmeric, and chili peppers, and sauté for 2 minutes while stirring constantly. Add the onion and cook another minute.

3. Add the potato, carrots, tomatoes, and green and red bell peppers. Cover with the remaining broth (if more liquid is needed, add additional broth or water). Stirring constantly, bring the mixture to a boil. Reduce the heat to medium–low and simmer uncovered for 20 minutes, or until the vegetables are cooked.

4. While the vegetables are cooking, bring the rice and water almost to a boil in a medium saucepan. Reduce the heat to low, cover, and simmer about 15 minutes, or until the rice is tender and the liquid is absorbed. Remove the pan from the heat and let stand for 5 minutes.

5. Mound the vegetables on a large serving platter. Surround the vegetables with a ring of rice, garnish with cilantro, and serve immediately.

Take a Chance:

• Use different vegetables. Try broccoli, zucchini, crookneck squash, or mushrooms.

• Add $1/4$ cup chopped walnuts to the garnish.

This one-dish meal is filled with savory vegetables and spices, and enlivened by onions, garlic, and chili peppers.

1 cup brown basmati rice

$1 1/4$ cups Vegetable Broth (page 59)

3 cloves garlic, finely chopped

$1/4$ teaspoon ground cumin

$1/4$ teaspoon ground coriander

$1/8$ teaspoon ground turmeric

2 serrano or Thai chili peppers, seeded and finely chopped

1 yellow or white onion, finely chopped

1 potato, cut into $1/2$-inch cubes

3 carrots, peeled and cut into $1/4$-inch slices

2 large tomatoes, seeded and coarsely chopped

1 green bell pepper, seeded and cut into $1/2$-inch pieces

1 red bell pepper, seeded and cut into $1/2$-inch pieces

$1 3/4$ cups water

3 tablespoons finely chopped cilantro

Vegetable Stew West Africa

This is a tasty version of one of our favorite West African recipes—Jollof Rice. It contains an interesting combination of colors and flavors.

3 tablespoons safflower oil

1 yellow or white onion, finely chopped

4 cloves garlic, finely chopped

2 jalapeño peppers, seeded and finely chopped

1/2 teaspoon thyme

1/4 teaspoon cinnamon

1 eggplant, cut into 1/2-inch pieces

8 ounces fresh or frozen spinach

1 yam, peeled and cut into 1/2-inch cubes

2 cups tomato sauce

1 cup rice

1/2 teaspoon freshly grated ginger

2 cups Vegetable Broth (page 59)

3 scallions, finely chopped

YIELD: 4 SERVINGS   PREPARATION TIME: 30 MINUTES

1. Place the oil in a large skillet over medium heat. Add the onion and garlic, and sauté for 5 minutes. Add the jalapeño peppers, thyme, and cinnamon, and continue to sauté for 2 minutes. Add the eggplant, spinach, and yam, and cook for 2 minutes. Reduce the heat to medium-low, and add 1 1/2 cups of the tomato sauce. Stir well, cover, and simmer for 20 minutes.

2. Place the remaining tomato sauce in a large saucepan. Add the rice and ginger, and stir over the heat until the rice begins to absorb the sauce. Add the broth, cover, and simmer over medium-low heat for 15 minutes, or until the rice is tender.

3. Spoon the rice into a serving bowl, top with the stew, and garnish with the scallions. Serve with Caesar Salad (page 43).

TAKE A CHANCE:

• After sautéing the spices, add 1/2 cup thinly sliced chicken or your favorite meat substitute, and sauté for 2 minutes.

• Add 1/2 cup chopped broccoli or sliced mushrooms.

• Use yucca (cassava) instead of the yam. Yucca is available in specialty and gourmet shops, and some grocery stores.

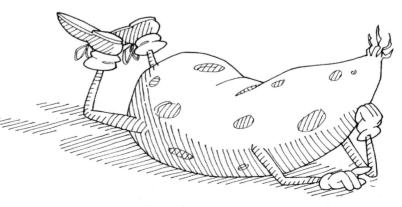

COUSCOUS with Summer Vegetables Morocco

1. Place ¼ cup of the broth in a large skillet over medium heat. Add the onions and sauté for 5 minutes. Add the garlic, coriander, cloves, cinnamon, and jalapeño peppers, and continue to sauté another minute. Add the zucchini, carrots, potatoes, bell peppers, eggplant, tomatoes, and another ¾ cup of the broth. Simmer uncovered for 15 minutes, adding more broth during cooking if the vegetables seem dry.

2. Bring the remaining cup of broth to boil in a small saucepan. Remove from the heat.

3. Place the couscous in a large bowl and add the warm broth. Cover the bowl and let stand for 10 minutes.

4. Fluff the couscous with a fork, then place it on a serving platter. Cover with the vegetables and serve immediately with Harissa Sauce (page 167) on the side.

TAKE A CHANCE:

• Add 1 cup tomato sauce to the vegetables.

• Add ½ cup raisins to the couscous.

• Use 1 or 2 small sweet potatoes instead of new potatoes.

*O*nions are used lavishly in Moroccan cooking. Here they are mixed with lightly cooked garden vegetables and served over couscous.

2 cups Vegetable Broth (page 59)

3 yellow or white onions, halved lengthwise then cut into ¼-inch pieces

4 cloves garlic, finely chopped

½ teaspoon ground coriander

⅛ teaspoon ground cloves

⅛ teaspoon ground cinnamon

2 jalapeño peppers, seeded and finely chopped

3 zucchini, cut into ½-inch slices

3 carrots, cut into ½-inch slices

4 new or red potatoes, cut into ½-inch cubes

2 green bell peppers, seeded and cut into ½-inch pieces

1 eggplant, peeled and cut into ½-inch cubes

3 tomatoes, seeded and coarsely chopped

2 cups couscous

Onion Leek Risotto Italy

Traditionally used in risotto, arborio rice is a staple of northern Italy. It is a starchy short grain rice that absorbs great quantities of liquid and turns creamy as it cooks. Although other rice can be used in this dish, arborio is preferred.

4 cups Vegetable Broth (page 59)

2 yellow or white onions, halved lengthwise then cut into $1/4$-inch pieces

2 tablespoons extra-virgin olive oil

3 leeks, white part only, thinly sliced

1 clove elephant garlic, finely minced

1 cup arborio rice

3 tablespoons finely chopped chives

YIELD: 4 SERVINGS   PREPARATION TIME: 45 MINUTES

1. Bring the broth to a boil in a large saucepan. Reduce the heat to low and continue to simmer.

2. Place the oil in another large saucepan over medium heat. Add the onions and sauté for 5 minutes. Add the leeks, garlic, and rice, and sauté another 3 minutes.

3. Stirring constantly, slowly add 1 cup of the broth to the rice. Continue stirring while the rice absorbs the liquid. Add another $1/2$ cup of the broth, and continue to stir until it is absorbed. Continue to add the remaining broth, $1/2$ cup at a time. This should take approximately 20 to 25 minutes.

4. When all of the broth has been added, continue to cook, stirring constantly, until the rice has a creamy texture and is cooked through. If you prefer a looser consistency, add a small quantity of broth before serving.

5. Garnish with the chives, and serve immediately. It is perfect alongside Broiled Onions with Raisin Sauce (page 136).

TAKE A CHANCE:

• Use 6 shallots, thinly sliced, instead of onions.

• Stir $1/4$ cup walnuts into the risotto before serving.

• When half the broth has been added to the rice, add 1 cup of vegetables, such as zucchini, mushrooms, tomatoes, or peas.

Trivia Tidbit

One head of elephant garlic can grow to be the size of an orange.

Baked Rice India

YIELD: 6 SERVINGS PREPARATION TIME: 45 MINUTES

1. Place the rice in a large bowl and cover with cold water. Rub the grains with your fingers then drain. Repeat this process 4 more times, then let the rice drain for 10 minutes.

2. In a 1½ quart saucepan, sauté the almonds in the oil for 5 minutes, or until they turn golden brown. With a slotted spoon, remove the almonds from the pan and drain on a paper towel. Set aside.

3. Add the onion, garlic, and jalapeños to the saucepan, and sauté for 2 minutes. Add the rice, ginger, and curry powder, and sauté another 5 minutes. Stir in the broth and continue to cook for 5 minutes, or until the top of the rice looks dry. Place the mixture in an ovenproof casserole dish and bake uncovered in a 325°F oven for 20 minutes, or until the rice is tender and all the liquid has been absorbed.

4. Garnish with the browned almonds and serve immediately with Hot Pickled Onions (page 156) and Onion & Garlic Chutney (page 175).

TAKE A CHANCE:

• Use walnuts instead of almonds.

• Add ¼ cup diced red bell pepper to the rice as it cooks.

Baked with onion and garlic, and made spicy with chili pepper, this rice adds an elegant touch to any meal.

3 cups long grain rice

¼ cup sliced almonds

3 tablespoons canola oil

1 yellow or white onion, halved lengthwise then cut into ¼-inch pieces

3 cloves garlic, finely chopped

2 Thai or serrano chili peppers, seeded and finely chopped

1 teaspoon freshly grated ginger

½ teaspoon curry powder

4 cups Chicken Broth (page 58)

¼ teaspoon freshly ground black pepper

Pasta with Garlic & Oil Italy

Classic "aglio e olio" combines the flavors of fresh garlic and extra-virgin olive oil. This dish is simple, elegant, and versatile, as the variations in the Take a Chance section show.

8 cloves garlic, finely chopped

$1/2$ cup extra-virgin olive oil

1 pound pasta, preferably spaghetti

$1/2$ teaspoon freshly ground black pepper

3 tablespoons finely chopped Italian parsley

YIELD: 4   PREPARATION TIME: 20 MINUTES

1. Mix together the garlic and olive oil in a small bowl and set aside.

2. Cook the pasta until it is firm but tender (al dente). Drain.

3. Add the garlic and oil mixture to the pasta and toss well.

4. Garnish with parsley and serve with Classic Garlic Bread (page 188).

TAKE A CHANCE:

• Sauté the garlic in the oil for 2 minutes before tossing with the pasta.

• Add $1/4$ teaspoon chopped fresh rosemary, or 10 chopped basil leaves to the garlic and oil mixture.

• Use Roasted Garlic (page 25) instead of raw.

• Add $1/2$ teaspoon crushed red pepper and/or 3 mashed anchovy fillets to the garlic and oil.

• Add 1 cup cooked broccoli or cauliflower florets to the pasta before tossing.

• Use $1/4$ cup olive oil and $1/4$ cup lemon juice instead of all olive oil.

• Use $1/2$ cup Garlic-Infused Olive Oil (page 174) or Pesto Sauce (page 172) instead of the garlic and oil.

Crispy Noodles with Garlic & Shallots Thailand

YIELD: 4 SERVINGS   PREPARATION TIME: 30 MINUTES

1. Place 2 tablespoons of the oil in a wok or large skillet over medium-high heat. Add half of the noodles and fry until crisp, about 2 minutes. With a slotted spoon, remove the noodles to a paper towel and drain. Repeat with the remaining noodles, adding more oil if necessary.

2. Add another tablespoon of oil to the wok and heat. Stir-fry the tofu for 10 minutes, or until the strips are brown. Place the tofu on paper toweling.

3. Add all of the sauce ingredients to the wok and mix well. Reduce the heat to medium and cook for 5 minutes. Return the cooked tofu to the wok, mix with the sauce, and cook another 5 minutes.

4. Place the remaining oil in a small pan over medium heat. Slowly add the egg mixture, stirring constantly until the egg is cooked dry and broken into pieces. Set aside.

5. Add the crispy noodles to the tofu and sauce, and cook for 1 minute.

6. Garnish with the scallions, bean sprouts, and cooked egg before serving.

TAKE A CHANCE:

• Add 1 ounce cooked ground chicken to the sauce.

• Add 3 seeded and finely chopped Thai chili peppers to the garnish.

• Serve with Pickled Garlic (page 158) on the side.

*G*arlic and shallots are used extensively in Thai cooking. Here they are paired with crispy noodles for a satisfying main meal.

4 tablespoons canola oil

4 ounces rice noodles*

8 ounces firm tofu, drained and cut into thin strips

$1/4$ cup egg substitute mixed with 1 tablespoon water

4 scallions, cut on an angle into $1/4$-inch pieces

1 ounce bean sprouts

Sauce

4 cloves garlic, finely chopped

4 shallots, finely chopped

2 tablespoons fish sauce (nuoc mam)*

$1/4$ cup fresh lemon juice

$1/4$ cup Vegetable Broth (page 59)

$1/2$ teaspoon chili powder

$1/4$ teaspoon freshly ground black pepper

* Available in Asian markets, gourmet shops, and some grocery stores.

Chapter 6

The Dinner Plate
Tasty Chicken and Fish

For those who enjoy chicken and fish in their diets, we present mouthwatering dishes that use garlic and onions as their secret to good taste. Flip through the following pages and see if your eye doesn't begin glancing at the refrigerator while your mind is making a mental inventory of the ingredients called for in the recipes. As your hand reaches for the garlic, you'll know you're hooked . . .

Spicy Chicken Fajitas Mexico

*O*nions and garlic add a flavorful bite to this spicy dish.

4 skinless, boneless, free-range chicken breasts, cut into 1/2-inch strips

2 teaspoons extra-virgin olive oil

1 green bell pepper, seeded and cut in 1/2 inch strips

1 red bell pepper, seeded and cut in 1/2-inch strips

2 poblano chili peppers, seeded and cut into 1/2-inch strips

8 flour tortillas

1 cup Salsa Cruda (page 22)

Marinade

1/4 cup lime juice

2 yellow or white onions, sliced lengthwise and cut in 1/2-inch pieces

2 cloves garlic, finely chopped

1/4 teaspoon cayenne pepper

1/4 teaspoon freshly ground black pepper

YIELD: 8 FAJITAS   PREPARATION TIME: 1 1/2 HOURS

1. Combine the marinade ingredients in a large bowl. Add the chicken and toss to coat. Cover and refrigerate for 1 hour.

2. Place the oil in a large skillet over medium heat. Add the green and red bell peppers and the poblano chilies, and sauté for 1 minute. Add the chicken and the marinade, and sauté for 5 minutes, or until the chicken is cooked through. Transfer to a serving bowl.

3. Spoon some of the filling on a tortilla, add some Salsa Cruda, and fold in half. Enjoy with a side dish of Black Bean Salad (page 49).

TAKE A CHANCE:

• Use strips of tofu instead of chicken.

Yassa Chicken Africa

YIELD: 4 SERVINGS   PREPARATION TIME: 6½ HOURS

1. Place the chicken in a large bowl and cover with the onions.

2. In a small bowl, combine the lemon juice and cayenne pepper, and pour over the onions. Cover and marinate in the refrigerator for at least 6 hours.

3. Place the onions and marinade in a skillet over medium heat, add the vegetable broth, and sauté for 5 minutes or until the onions are soft. Add the chicken and continue to sauté for 10 minutes, or until the chicken is cooked.

4. Serve immediately with Spicy Mashed Potato Salad (page 54).

TAKE A CHANCE:

• Leave the chicken breasts whole and cook on the barbecue or in the oven. Pour the cooked marinade over the chicken before serving.

*I*n this dish, the onions and lemon combine for a tart, spicy taste.

4 skinless, boneless free-range chicken breasts, cut into ½-inch strips

2 yellow or white onions, thinly sliced

½ cup fresh lemon juice

½ teaspoon cayenne pepper

4 tablespoons Vegetable Broth (page 59)

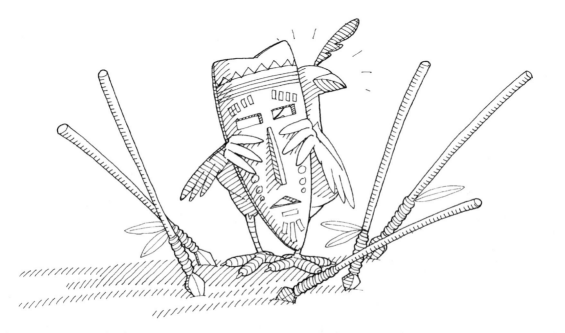

Chicken Stew Brazil

*B*ecause *they were easy to carry and grow, garlic and onions were common items brought by explorers to the New World. Today, these hardy alliums are staples of the South American cuisine. This delicious stew comes from the Brazilian province of Bahia.*

1/4 cup Chicken Broth (page 58)

2 yellow or white onions, thinly sliced

4 cloves garlic, chopped

3 jalapeño peppers, seeded and chopped

2 tomatoes, peeled, seeded and chopped

1/2 cup finely chopped cilantro

3-pound free-range chicken, skinned and cut into 8 pieces

2 cups coconut milk

1/2 cup finely ground dried shrimp* (optional)

1 cup ground roasted peanuts

1/4 teaspoon freshly ground black pepper

* Available at Latin American and Asian markets.

YIELD: 4 SERVINGS PREPARATION TIME: 1 HOUR

1. Place the broth in a large skillet over medium heat. Add the onions and sauté for 1 minute. Add the garlic and jalapeño peppers, and sauté another minute. Add the tomatoes and cilantro, and simmer 10 minutes more.

2. Add the chicken to the skillet and simmer uncovered for 30 minutes, or until the chicken is very tender and falling off the bone. If necessary, add additional broth or water to the skillet to keep the ingredients moist. Transfer the chicken to a cutting board and allow to cool.

3. Reduce the heat to low, and add the coconut milk, shrimp, peanuts, and black pepper to the skillet. Stirring occasionally, cook the sauce 10 minutes or until it becomes thick.

4. While the sauce cooks, debone the chicken. When the sauce has thickened, add the chicken and heat through.

5. Serve immediately alongside Mashed Potatoes with Onion & Lemon (page 128).

TAKE A CHANCE:

• Add 8 ounces of trimmed mushrooms to the stew.

• Use the thinly sliced white portion of 3 medium leeks instead of the onion.

• Omit the dried shrimp.

• Use tofu instead of chicken. Cut 1 pound of firm tofu into 1/2-inch slices and simmer in the onion mixture. Remove the simmered tofu and cut it into small cubes. Return the cubes to the skillet when the sauce has thickened.

Chicken Adobo Phillipines

YIELD: 4 SERVINGS   PREPARATION TIME: 2 HOURS

1. Combine the garlic and black pepper in a small bowl.

2. Rub each piece of chicken with the garlic mixture and place in a large bowl. Pour the soy sauce and vinegar over the chicken, cover the bowl, and marinate in the refrigerator for 1 hour, turning the chicken at least once.

3. Place the chicken and the marinade in a large skillet over medium-low heat. Simmer gently for 45 minutes.

4. Transfer the chicken to a broiling pan, and broil for 5 minutes on each side, or until the chicken is browned.

5. Bring the marinade to a boil and cook until it is reduced by half.

6. Pour the sauce over the chicken and serve immediately with Yucca in Garlic Sauce (page 151).

TAKE A CHANCE:

• Use fresh lemon juice instead of vinegar.

• Barbecue the chicken instead of broiling it.

• If the reduced-sodium soy sauce is still too salty, reduce the amount and add an equal amount of fresh lemon juice.

Filipino cuisine is a curious blend of many cultures. The use of garlic and vinegar gives this dish a Spanish flare, while the soy sauce adds a Far Eastern influence. Although deep-frying the chicken in lard is the traditional cooking method for Chicken Adobo, we have found simmering to be a healthier—and just as flavorful—choice.

Cloves from 1 head of garlic, crushed

1 teaspoon freshly ground black pepper

2^1/$_2$-pound free-range chicken, skinned and cut into 8 pieces.

1 cup reduced-sodium shoyu or tamari soy sauce

1 cup distilled white vinegar

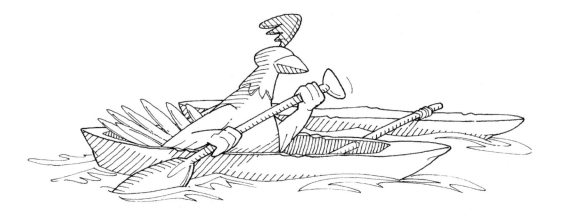

Chicken Breasts with Garlic & Shallots Cuba

We've added shallots to this piquant dish of chicken with garlic sauce.

4 skinless, boneless free-range chicken breasts

2 tablespoons extra-virgin olive oil

6 cloves garlic, thinly sliced

2 large shallots, thinly sliced

1/2 cup dry white wine

1/4 cup fresh cilantro

YIELD: 4 SERVINGS   PREPARATION TIME: 25 MINUTES

1. Place the oil in a skillet over medium heat. Add the chicken and sauté for 3 minutes on each side. Remove the chicken to a warm plate and set aside.

2. Add the garlic, shallots, and wine to the skillet, and sauté for 2 minutes. Return the chicken to the skillet and continue to cook for 10 minutes, or until the chicken is cooked through. Add the cilantro and stir.

3. Place the cooked breasts on a platter, cover with the sauce, and serve alongside Roasted Vidalias (page 135).

TAKE A CHANCE:

• Add 3 seeded, diced jalapeño peppers to the sauce.

• Add 3 tablespoons fresh lemon juice to the sauce just before serving.

FREE-RANGE CHICKENS

Chickens have been fully domesticated for at least 4,000 years. Developed mainly from a red jungle fowl of Southeast Asia, chickens have been raised for food and sport, and for the use of their eggs and feathers.

Due to the growing demand of chickens for food, many farmers raise large numbers of birds under cramped conditions and feed them hormones, which increase their size and weight. Recently, a health-conscious public has become aware of these farming methods and is demanding healthier, hormone-free fowl. As a result, an increasing number of farmers are raising free-range chickens.

Free-range chickens are able to roam freely under spacious conditions and are fed hormone-free organic grains. Because they are not given hormones, these chickens take longer to mature. Free-range chickens may be costlier than others, but they are also tastier and healthier. You can buy free-range chickens in gourmet shops, natural foods stores, and a growing number of supermarkets and butcher shops.

Chicken Paprika Hungary

YIELD: 4 SERVINGS   PREPARATION TIME: 45 MINUTES

1. Place the oil in a large skillet over medium heat. Add the onion and sauté for 2 minutes. Add the garlic and paprika, and sauté another minute. Add the chicken and sauté 5 minutes on each side.

2. Reduce the heat to low, add the broth, and simmer covered for 25 minutes, or until the chicken is cooked. Transfer the chicken to a plate. Add the arrowroot to the skillet and stir constantly for 5 minutes, or until the liquid begins to thicken. Return the chicken to the skillet and heat through.

3. Remove from the heat, stir in the sour cream, and serve immediately with Garlic Green Beans (page 125).

TAKE A CHANCE:

• Use 4 large shallots instead of the onion.

The Hungarian countryside is dotted with fields of sweet red pepper plants. Paprika—a mild powdered seasoning made from these plants—is used in this traditional Hungarian dish.

2 tablespoons canola oil

2 onions, finely chopped

3 cloves garlic, finely chopped

2 tablespoons paprika (preferably Hungarian)

3-pound free-range chicken, skinned and cut into 8 pieces

1 cup Chicken Broth (page 58)

2 tablespoons arrowroot

$^1/_2$ cup nonfat sour cream

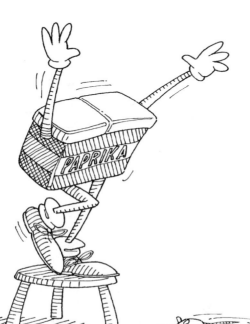

Hot Island Chicken Caribbean

Hot chili peppers mixed with cool onions and garlic will have you coming back for second helpings of this island treat.

2 tablespoons canola oil

4 skinless, boneless free-range chicken breasts, cut into large pieces

1/4 cup finely chopped yellow or white onion

2 habañero chili peppers, seeded and finely chopped

4 cloves garlic, finely chopped

2 tablespoons finely chopped fresh cilantro

1/4 teaspoon ground cloves

1/4 teaspoon freshly ground black pepper

Juice of 2 limes

4 scallions, finely chopped

YIELD: 4 SERVINGS   PREPARATION TIME: 20 MINUTES

1. Place the oil in a large skillet over medium heat. Add the chicken and sauté for 2 minutes. Add all of the remaining ingredients, except the lime juice and scallions, and sauté for 5 minutes, or until the chicken is cooked through. Add the lime juice and stir well.

2. Garnish the chicken with scallions, and serve immediately with Caesar Salad (page 43).

TAKE A CHANCE:

• To cut the heat, use 3 or 4 jalapeño or serrano chili peppers instead of the habañeros.

• Leave the chicken breasts whole. Mix the chili peppers, onion, garlic, cilantro, cloves, and black pepper together. Cut deep slashes in the chicken breasts and fill with the mixture. Sauté or bake the chicken until cooked.

• Use ground cinnamon instead of cloves.

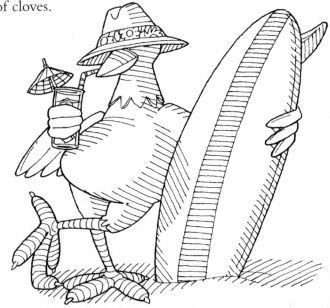

Spicy Sweet Chicken Israel

YIELD: 4 SERVINGS   PREPARATION TIME: 1½ HOURS

1. Place the oil in a large skillet over medium heat. Add the chicken and sauté 5 minutes on each side, or until golden brown.

2. While the chicken cooks, combine the orange juice, honey, ginger, nutmeg, and black pepper in a small bowl and stir well. Set aside.

3. Coat a 3-quart ovenproof casserole dish with nonstick spray. Place half the onions on the bottom of the dish, then add the sautéed chicken and olives. Pour half the orange juice mixture over the chicken, and top with the remaining onions. Pour the remaining juice over the onions. Cover and bake in a 350°F oven for 30 minutes.

4. In a small bowl, dissolve the arrowroot in a tablespoon of water. Add the mixture to the chicken and continue cooking another 30 minutes, or until the chicken is cooked and the juice mixture is slightly thickened.*

5. Garnish the chicken with orange sections and serve with Stewed Onions, Eggplant, & Tomatoes (page 149).

* If the juice mixture is not thick enough when the chicken is done, remove the chicken from the casserole dish and set it aside. In a saucepan on the stove, bring the liquid to a boil, stirring constantly until it thickens.

TAKE A CHANCE:

• Use lemon juice and lemon sections instead of the orange.

*O*nions and olives combine with sweet oranges and flavorful spices in this delicious casserole.

2 tablespoons canola oil

3-pound free-range chicken, skinned and cut into 8 pieces

¾ cup fresh orange juice

2 teaspoons honey

¼ teaspoon freshly grated ginger

⅛ teaspoon nutmeg

¼ teaspoon freshly ground black pepper

2 yellow or white onions, thinly sliced

12 brine-cured black olives

2 teaspoons arrowroot

1 large orange, peeled and cut into sections

Vindaloo India

In spite of its lengthy marinating time, this chicken dish is quick and easy to prepare. It is a perfect entrée to serve guests.

2¹/₂-pound free-range chicken, skinned and cut into 8 pieces

2 teaspoons canola oil

2 onions, finely chopped

1 bay leaf

Marinade

¹/₂ cup distilled white vinegar

2 teaspoons ground coriander

2 teaspoons turmeric

2 teaspoons ground cumin

1 teaspoon dry mustard

¹/₂ teaspoon cayenne pepper

YIELD: 4 SERVINGS   PREPARATION TIME: 7 HOURS

1. Combine the marinade ingredients in a small bowl.

2. Place the chicken in a shallow dish and cover with the marinade. Cover the dish and refrigerate 6 hours, turning the pieces at least 3 times.

3. Place the oil in a large skillet over medium heat. Add the onion and bay leaf, and sauté for 10 minutes. Reduce the heat to medium-low and add the chicken and marinade. Cover and simmer for 35 minutes, or until the chicken is cooked through.

4. Serve immediately with Crunchy Cucumber Salad (page 48) and Onion & Garlic Chutney (page 175)

TAKE A CHANCE:

• Use 3 seeded, chopped serrano or Thai chili peppers instead of the cayenne pepper.

• Add 2 teaspoons freshly grated ginger to the spices.

• Use shrimp instead of chicken. Reduce the marinating time to 1 hour, and reduce the cooking time to 5 minutes or until the shrimp turn pink.

Doro Wat **Ethiopia**

1. Place the chicken in a large dish and cover with the Berbere Sauce. Cover and refrigerate for 1 hour.

2. Place the oil in a large skillet over medium heat. Add the onion and sauté for 3 minutes. Add the garlic, black pepper, and nutmeg, and sauté another 2 minutes. Add the marinated chicken and water. Bring the ingredients to a boil, then reduce the heat to medium-low. Cook covered for 40 minutes, or until the chicken is very tender and starts falling off the bone.

3. Serve immediately with Lime-Marinated Onion Rings (page 157) and a side dish of Spicy Steamed Vegetables (page 144).

TAKE A CHANCE:

- Add 1 teaspoon of cayenne pepper and 1 tablespoon paprika to the sautéing garlic. For a five-alarm version, add a tablespoon of each.

This delicious chicken stew adds a double dose of onions and garlic—one in the delicious Berbere sauce and another in the stew itself.

2½-pound free-range chicken, skinned and cut into 8 pieces

½ cup Berbere Sauce (page 166)

2 tablespoons canola oil

1 yellow or white onion, finely chopped

4 cloves garlic, finely chopped

½ teaspoon freshly ground black pepper

⅛ teaspoon ground nutmeg

1¾ cup water

Chicken with 40 Cloves of Garlic France

arlic is the foundation of Provençal cuisine. When roasted with the chicken in this dish, the garlic mellows and fills the kitchen with a wonderful bouquet.

3-pound free-range chicken

$^1/_2$ teaspoon coarsely chopped fresh rosemary

$^1/_2$ teaspoon coarsely chopped fresh thyme

4 fresh sage leaves, coarsely chopped

4 tablespoons coarsely chopped parsley

40 cloves garlic (about 4 heads), peeled

3 tablespoons Chicken Broth (page 58)

3 tablespoons extra-virgin olive oil

$^1/_2$ teaspoon freshly ground black pepper

YIELD: 4 SERVINGS   PREPARATION TIME: 1 $^1/_2$ HOURS

1. Place the chicken in a roasting pan. In a small bowl, combine half of the rosemary, thyme, sage, and parsley, and 6 cloves of garlic. Place the mixture inside the chicken.

2. In another bowl, combine the broth, olive oil, and black pepper with the remaining rosemary, thyme, sage, and parsley. Pour this mixture over the chicken. Surround the chicken with the remaining garlic cloves.

3. Cover and bake in a 350°F oven for 1$^1/_4$ hours, or until the chicken is cooked through.

4. Transfer the chicken to a serving platter and keep it warm. Spoon the cooking juices into a gravy boat after skimming off the fat. Place the roasted cloves on a dish.

5. Serve the chicken with the sauce, the roasted garlic, and a side dish of Fresh Peas with Pearl Onions (page 137).

TAKE A CHANCE:

• Use a clay cooker instead of a roasting pan to cook the chicken.

• For a milder taste, use 2 cloves of elephant garlic instead of 40 cloves of regular garlic.

• Spread the roasted garlic cloves on crusty slices of French bread.

Baked Fish with Onions & Tomato Sauce Greece

YIELD: 4 SERVINGS   PREPARATION TIME: 45 MINUTES

1. Place the broth in a large skillet over medium heat. Add the onion and sauté another minute. Add the lemon juice, tomato sauce, and cloves, and cook 5 minutes.

2. Place 3 tablespoons of the sauce in the bottom of an oven-proof baking dish. Add the fish and sprinkle with black pepper. Pour the remaining sauce over the fish, cover, and bake at 350°F for 35 minutes or until the fish is white and flaky. Baste the fish several times as it bakes.

3. Garnish with parsley and serve immediately alongside Garlic-Stuffed Artichokes (page 124).

TAKE A CHANCE:

• Add 1 teaspoon grated lemon rind to the fish as it bakes.

• Omit the tomato sauce from Step 1, and spread 1 cup of Skordalia (page 168) over the fish before garnishing with parsley.

*F*resh fish that is caught in the waters off Greek seaside resorts is commonly baked with onions and garlic in tomato sauce. Serve this Mediterranean classic with plenty of fresh crusty bread to soak up all the flavorful sauce.

$^1/_4$ cup Vegetable Broth (page 59)

2 medium yellow or white onions, thinly sliced

4 cloves garlic, crushed

$^1/_4$ cup fresh lemon juice

2 cups tomato sauce

2 whole cloves

1 pound white fish fillets, such as cod

$^1/_4$ teaspoon freshly ground pepper

2 tablespoons fresh chopped parsley

Trivia Tidbit

When using herbs, it is generally better to use fresh rather than dried. However, when dried is all that is available, use the following conversion:

1 tablespoon fresh herb = 1 teaspoon dried.

Creole Fish & Shrimp United States

Creole food originated in New Orleans and is influenced by both French and Spanish cuisines. Onions and garlic blend with green peppers and tomatoes to help counterbalance the heat of the cayenne pepper.

3 tablespoons extra-virgin olive oil

2 yellow or white onions, finely chopped

3 cloves garlic, finely chopped

2 teaspoons cayenne pepper

1/4 teaspoon dried thyme

1/2 teaspoon freshly ground black pepper

2 celery ribs, leaves included, coarsely chopped

1 green bell pepper, coarsely chopped

12 ounces white fish, such as cod, sole, or flounder

8 ounces medium shrimp, cleaned

1 teaspoon filé powder*

2 scallions, finely chopped

* A traditional thickening agent used in Creole cooking, filé (powdered sassafras leaves) is available at most gourmet shops.

1. Place the oil in a large skillet over medium heat. Add the onions and garlic, and sauté for 1 minute. Add the cayenne pepper, thyme, and black pepper, and continue to sauté another minute.

2. Add the celery, bell pepper, and tomatoes, and cook another 10 minutes.

3. Add the fish and cook 5 minutes, then add the shrimp and cook another 5 minutes.

4. Remove the skillet from the heat and stir in the filé powder. Garnish with scallions and serve immediately with plain rice and a simple salad dressed with Garlic Lemon Vinaigrette (page 159).

Take a Chance:

• Use 2 teaspoons of hot sauce instead of or in addition to the cayenne pepper.

• Omit the shrimp and increase the amount of white fish to 1 1/2 pounds.

Curried Prawns Malaysia

YIELD: 4 SERVINGS   PREPARATION TIME: 20 MINUTES

1. Place the oil in a large skillet or wok over medium heat. Add the onion and garlic, and sauté for 2 minutes. Add the chili peppers, ginger, and turmeric, and continue to cook 3 minutes more.

2. Add the coriander and water, and cook another minute. If the mixture is too dry, add another teaspoon of water. Stir in the shrimp, green beans, and vinegar. Cook 5 minutes or until the shrimp turn pink.

3. Remove the chili peppers and place the shrimp in a serving bowl. Serve immediately with Fried Rice (page 85).

TAKE A CHANCE:

• For a hotter taste, use dried chili peppers instead of fresh.

• Use lemon juice instead of vinegar.

This exotic shrimp dish is surprisingly quick and easy to make.

2 tablespoons canola oil

2 cups finely chopped yellow or white onion

3 cloves garlic, finely chopped

4 whole Thai or serrano chili peppers

1 teaspoon freshly grated ginger

$1/4$ teaspoon turmeric

2 teaspoons water

$1/2$ teaspoon ground coriander

1 pound medium shrimp, cleaned

1 cup cooked green beans

2 teaspoons vinegar

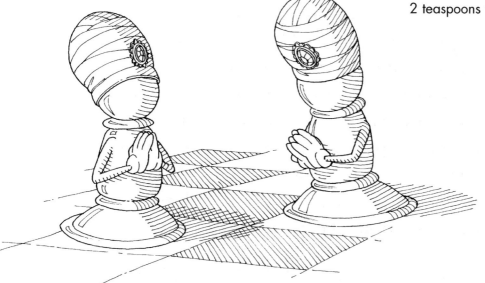

Shrimp Scampi Italy

Saturated with garlic, these luscious shrimp won't last long on your plate.

2 tablespoons soy margarine

2 tablespoons Vegetable Broth (page 59)

6 cloves garlic, crushed

1/2 cup dry white wine

2 tablespoons tomato paste

1 1/2 pounds shrimp, cleaned

2 tablespoons finely chopped fresh parsley

YIELD: 4 SERVINGS   PREPARATION TIME: 10 MINUTES

1. Place the margarine and broth in a skillet over medium heat. Add the garlic and sauté for 30 seconds, then add the wine and tomato paste and continue cooking while stirring constantly. Add the shrimp and continue to cook for 5 minutes, or until the shrimp turns pink.

2. Garnish with parsley and serve immediately over plain rice or pasta.

TAKE A CHANCE:

• Serve the scampi over Pasta with Garlic & Oil (page 100).

• For a milder taste, use 2 cloves of elephant garlic instead of regular cloves.

• Add 1 finely chopped shallot, and sauté with garlic.

• Add 2 teaspoons crushed red pepper, and sauté with the garlic.

Trivia Tidbit

Many recipes call for small amounts of tomato paste. Instead of opening a whole can and discarding the rest, or forgetting about it somewhere in the back of the refrigerator, look for tomato paste that comes in a tube. Simply open the tube, squeeze out the needed amount, and close it back up. Refrigerated, the paste will keep a long time. Also look for tubes of pesto sauce and anchovy paste.

Shrimp with Three Onions Thailand

YIELD: 4 SERVINGS   PREPARATION TIME: 20 MINUTES

1. Heat the broth, lemon juice, and fish sauce in a large skillet over high heat for 1 minute. Add the chili powder and continue to cook for another minute, then add the shrimp and cook another 3 minutes. Add the onions and shallots and continue cooking for 2 minutes, or until the shrimp turn pink.

2. Remove the skillet from the heat and stir in the scallions.

3. Serve immediately alongside Cabbage Salad with Peppered Onions (page 42).

TAKE A CHANCE:

• Use 2 or 3 seeded, finely chopped Thai peppers instead of chili powder.

These savory shrimp are blanketed under three varieties of onion.

1/4 cup Vegetable Broth (page 59)

1/4 cup fresh lemon juice

3 tablespoons fish sauce (nuoc mam)*

1 teaspoon chili powder

1 pound medium shrimp, cleaned

1 yellow or white onion, finely chopped

2 shallots, coarsely chopped

3 scallions, cut diagonally into 1-inch pieces

* Available in Asian markets, gourmet shops, and some grocery stores.

Broiled Tuna with Garlic & Shallot Marinade Cuba

*F*resh tuna is enhanced with a delicate marinade in this sensational dish.

1 1/2 pounds tuna fillets

Marinade

1/2 cup fresh lemon juice

2 tablespoons extra-virgin olive oil

3 cloves garlic, finely chopped

2 shallots, finely chopped

3 tablespoons finely chopped cilantro

1/4 teaspoon cayenne pepper

YIELD: 4 SERVINGS   PREPARATION TIME: 1 1/4 HOURS

1. Place the tuna in a large flat pan a single layer.

2. Combine the marinade ingredients and pour it over the fish. Cover and refrigerate for 1 hour.

3. Transfer the fish and marinade to a broiler pan that has been coated with nonstick spray. Broil the fish at 450°F for 5 minutes on each side, or until the fish is cooked.

4. Serve immediately alongside Yucca in Garlic Sauce (page 151).

TAKE A CHANCE:

• Reduce the lemon juice to 1/4 cup and add 1/4 cup lime juice.

• Add 3 seeded and chopped jalapeño or serrano chili peppers to the marinade.

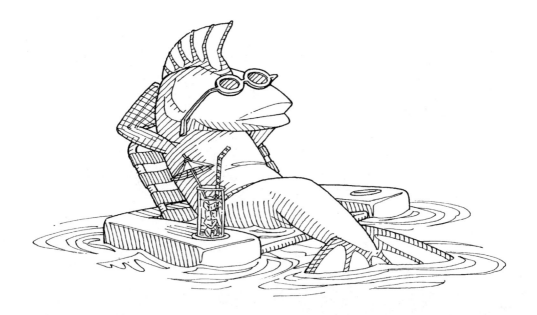

Salmon Kebabs with Garlic Chili Sauce Turkey / Thailand

YIELD: 4 SERVINGS PREPARATION TIME: 45 MINUTES

1. Place the fish in a medium bowl and add the lemon juice and chili sauce. Cover and refrigerate for 30 minutes.

2. Alternate threading the fish, onion, and green pepper on metal skewers (or bamboo skewers that have been soaked in water for 30 minutes).

3. Broil the kebabs at 450°F for 5 minutes per side, or until the fish is cooked through.

4. Garnish with cilantro and serve immediately with Pickled Garlic (page 158) and an Onion Tart (page 146).

TAKE A CHANCE:

• Use shark or tuna instead of salmon.

• Use whole pearl onions instead of the cut onions.

• Grill the kebabs on the barbecue instead of broiling them.

• Omit the Garlic Chili Sauce. After grilling, serve the kebabs with Garlic Shoyu Dip (page 160).

Here's an example of international cuisine at its best. We take a classic Turkish kebab and substitute salmon for the traditional lamb. Then we coat the fish with Thailand-influenced garlic sauce.

1 pound salmon steaks, boned and cut into $1/2$-inch pieces

4 teaspoons fresh lemon juice

1 recipe Garlic Chili Sauce (page 168)

1 yellow or white onion, quartered

1 green bell pepper, seeded and cut into 1-inch pieces

2 tablespoons chopped cilantro

Chapter 7

Cry-Your-Eyes-Out Vegetables

Talk about tear-jerkers. Just try any one these veggie dishes and you'll cry your eyes out with delight. Then you and your guests will cry again when there are no leftovers. Heartbreaking, yes, but you can always make more (or make double portions to begin with) whether it be for that special dinner party or for a cozy meal with your allium-loving family.

Garlic-Stuffed Artichokes Italy

Bursting with pungent garlic and sweet parsley, these artichokes make a prefect first course or light luncheon entrée.

4 artichokes

2 heads garlic, peeled and finely chopped

1 cup finely minced fresh parsley

1¼ cups dry white wine

¾ cup fresh lemon juice

¼ cup finely chopped yellow or white onion

10 whole black peppercorns

2 teaspoons extra-virgin olive oil

YIELD: 4 SERVINGS PREPARATION TIME: 1 HOUR

1. Place each artichoke on its side and carefully slice about ¹/₂ inch from the top. Remove the stems from the bottoms, so the artichokes can sit upright. Pull the leaves apart and remove the thorny center (choke) with a spoon and discard.

2. Place a layer of garlic in the cavity of each artichoke, then top with a layer of parsley. Repeat the layering until each cavity is full. Be sure to end with a layer of garlic.

3. Arrange the artichokes in a single layer in a large, deep skillet. Add the wine, lemon juice, onion, and peppercorns to the skillet. Cover and simmer over medium–low heat for 30 minutes, or until the artichokes are tender. (When you can easily pull a leaf from the center of the artichoke, it is cooked.)

4. Drizzle the olive oil over the artichokes and serve immediately.

TAKE A CHANCE:

• Add 4 mashed anchovy fillets to the wine and lemon juice mixture.

Trivia Tidbit

Garlic breath can be controlled by eating fresh lemon slices or parsley at the end of a meal. But the most effective way to conquer garlic breath is to feed lots of it to everyone!

Steamed Aspargus with Shallots France / United States

YIELD: 4   PREPARATION TIME: 20 MINUTES

1. Steam the asparagus for 20 minutes, or until tender. Do not overcook.

2. Transfer the asparagus to a serving platter, top with Shallot Spread, and serve immediately.

TAKE A CHANCE:

• Garnish with slivers of roasted red pepper.

• Serve cold with Garlic Lemon Vinaigrette (page 159).

*T*ender asparagus spears are enhanced by sweet shallots in this dish.

1 pound asparagus spears, ends trimmed

3 tablespoons Shallot Spread (page 171)

Garlic Green Beans Greece / France

YIELD: 4 SERVINGS   PREPARATION TIME: 20 MINUTES

1. Bring 4 quarts of water to boil in a large kettle, add the green beans, and cook for 2 minutes. Drain.

2. Melt the margarine in a large skillet over medium heat. Add the garlic and sauté for 1 minute. Toss in the green beans and continue to cook for 3 minutes. The beans should be very crisp yet tender.

3. Transfer the beans to a serving bowl and enjoy immediately.

TAKE A CHANCE:

• Add 8 pearl onions to the boiling water along with the green beans.

*C*ooked twice, these beans have a heady garlic taste and aroma.

1 pound green beans, trimmed

1 tablespoon soy margarine

6 cloves garlic, finely chopped

Mess O' Onions United States

Our love of the allium family led us to create this pungent, tasty treat. Try spreading a mess of these onions on crackers, dark rye bread, or baked potatoes. They are also delicious to eat all by themselves.

2 tablespoons extra-virgin olive oil

2 tablespoons soy margarine

2 yellow or white onions, thinly sliced

6 scallions, thinly sliced

3 shallots, coarsely chopped

1/2 teaspoon freshly ground black pepper

1 teaspoon minced fresh chives

YIELD: 4 SERVINGS   PREPARATION TIME: 30 MINUTES

1. Place the oil and margarine in a skillet over low heat. When the margarine has melted, add the onions and sauté for 20 minutes, stirring occasionally until they just begin to brown. Add the scallions and shallots, and sauté for an additional 5 minutes, stirring occasionally.

2. Remove the skillet from the heat, add the black pepper, and mix thoroughly.

3. Place in a serving bowl, garnish with chives, and serve immediately.

TAKE A CHANCE:

• Add a dash of cinnamon before serving.

• For a mild garlic taste, add a minced clove of elephant garlic.

Trivia Tidbit

You can remove the smell of garlic and onions from your hands by rubbing them with a slice of fresh tomato or lemon.

Garlic Mashed Potatoes France

YIELD: 4 SERVINGS   PREPARATION TIME: 30 MINUTES

1. Place the potatoes in a large pot and cover with water. Cover the pot and bring to a boil, then reduce the heat to medium. Simmer the potatoes until they are tender. Drain.

2. While your food processor is running, drop in the garlic cloves through the access opening in the cover, and finely chop. Add the potatoes and broth, and process until the potatoes are smooth. Add more broth if the potatoes are too dry.

3. Spoon the potatoes into a serving bowl, garnish with chives, and serve immediately.

TAKE A CHANCE:

- For a milder taste, boil the garlic with the potatoes.
- Use 2 heads Roasted Garlic (page 25) instead of raw.
- For a Russian version of these potatoes, omit the broth and add $^3/_4$ cup nonfat sour cream.

From its humble beginning in the Peruvian highlands, the potato has grown to be a versatile ingredient in cuisines throughout the world. In this dish, the French have raised simple mashed potatoes to new heights by pairing them with one of our favorite flavors—garlic.

4 baking potatoes, peeled and quartered

10 cloves garlic

$^1/_2$ cup Vegetable Broth (page 59)

2 tablespoons finely chopped garlic chives

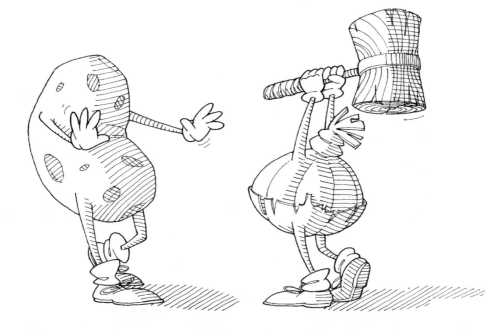

Mashed Potatoes with Onion & Lemon Peru

Peruvians mix Old World and New by combining lemon and onions with their own potatoes and chili peppers.

4 baking potatoes, quartered

1 yellow or white onion

2 jalapeño chili peppers, seeded and quartered

$1/2$ cup fresh lemon juice

2 scallions, finely chopped

2 hard boiled eggs, quartered

$1/4$ cup pitted black or green olives

YIELD: 4 SERVINGS   PREPARATION TIME: 30 MINUTES

1. Place the potatoes in a large pot and cover with water. Cover the pot and bring to a boil, then reduce the heat to medium. Simmer the potatoes until they are tender. Drain.

2. In a food processor, finely chop the onion and chili peppers. Add the potatoes and lemon juice, and process until the potatoes are smooth. Add more lemon juice or Vegetable Broth (page 59) if the potatoes are too dry.

3. Spoon the potatoes onto a serving platter and garnish with scallions. Surround the potatoes with the eggs and olives. Serve immediately.

TAKE A CHANCE:

• Add $1/2$ cup grated Muenster or Monterey Jack cheese to the blender.

• Use 2 teaspoons crushed red pepper instead of the jalapeños.

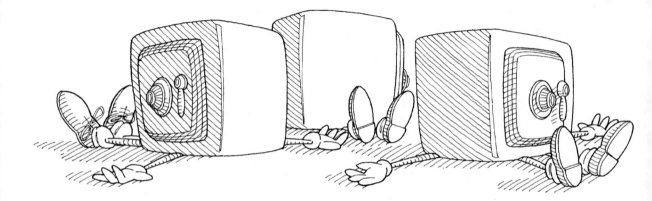

Mashed Potatoes & Leeks Ireland

YIELD: 4 SERVINGS PREPARATION TIME: 25 MINUTES

1. Melt the margarine in a skillet over medium heat. Add the leeks and black pepper, and sauté for 10 minutes. Remove from the heat and set aside.

2. Place the potatoes in a large pot and cover with water. Cover the pot and bring to a boil, then reduce the heat to medium. Simmer the potatoes until they are tender. Drain.

3. Place the cooked potatoes in a food processor, add the milk, and blend until smooth. Add more milk if the potatoes are too dry.

4. Transfer the potatoes to a large serving bowl and fold in the leeks. Serve immediately.

TAKE A CHANCE:

• Instead of milk, use $3/4$ cup plain nonfat yogurt or a mixture of yogurt and whipped tofu.

*M*ild and sweet, leeks go very well with mashed potatoes.

2 tablespoons soy margarine

4 leeks, trimmed, halved lengthwise, and thinly sliced

$1/8$ teaspoon freshly ground black pepper

4 baking potatoes, quartered

$3/4$ cup skim milk

Trivia Tidbit

The French refer to leeks as "asparagus for the poor."

Rumbledethumps Scotland

This hearty dish is a delightful but unlikely combination of mashed potatoes, onions, and shredded cabbage.

2 1/2 cups shredded cabbage

3 baking potatoes, peeled, quartered, and boiled

1/2 cup skim milk

2 teaspoons soy margarine

1 teaspoon canola oil

1 1/2 yellow or white onions, finely chopped

2 teaspoons finely chopped fresh parsley

1/8 teaspoon freshly ground black pepper

1/2 cup shredded lowfat cheddar cheese

YIELD: 4 SERVINGS   PREPARATION TIME: 1 HOUR

1. Bring a large pot of water to a boil. Add the cabbage and blanch for 1 minute. Drain and set aside.

2. Place the potatoes, milk, and margarine in a food processor, and blend until smooth. Add more milk if the potatoes are too dry.

3. Spoon the potatoes into a large bowl and mix in the cabbage.

4. Place the oil in a small skillet over medium heat. Add the onions and sauté for 5 minutes. Add the sautéed onions to the potatoes, along with the parsley and black pepper. Mix well.

5. Spray a 2-quart ovenproof casserole dish with nonstick cooking spray. Spoon the potato mixture into the casserole, smooth it evenly, and top with the cheddar cheese. Bake in a 350°F oven for 35 minutes, or until the potatoes are heated through and the cheese turns a golden brown.

6. Serve immediately.

TAKE A CHANCE:

• Use Monterey Jack cheese instead of cheddar.

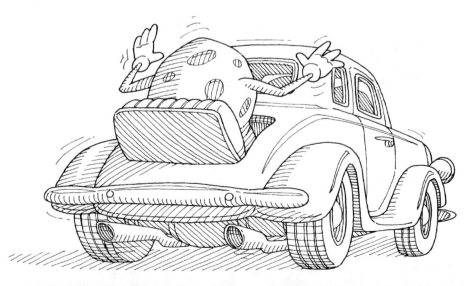

Baked Potatoes with Garlic Chives United States

Yield: 4 Servings   Preparation Time: 1 Hour

1. Pierce the potatoes and place them on a baking sheet. Bake in a 350°F oven for 1 hour, or until the potatoes are tender.

2. Place the cottage cheese in a food processor and blend until smooth.

3. Split the baked potatoes in half, top with the whipped cottage cheese, and garnish with garlic chives. Serve immediately.

Take a Chance:

- Use nonfat sour cream (which does not need to be whipped) instead of cottage cheese.

- Use Creamy Roasted Garlic Sauce (page 169) instead of cottage cheese.

- Add 1 chopped shallot to the cottage cheese before whipping.

Not only simple but elegant as well, a baked potato goes with almost any meal. The potato itself is very healthful—but watch out for those high-fat toppings. Instead of using butter, margarine, or sour cream, we have crowned these potatoes with whipped nonfat cottage cheese.

4 baking potatoes, scrubbed

3/4 cup nonfat cottage cheese

2 tablespoons finely chopped garlic chives

Trivia Tidbit

In the late 1700s, a book entitled *A Treatise of Gardening by a Citizen of Virginia* by John Randolph, recommended the use of chives because they do not affect the breath.

Stovies Scotland

YIELD: 4 SERVINGS   PREPARATION TIME: 35 MINUTES

This tasty Scottish side dish alternates slices of potato and onion with fresh herbs.

8 large red potatoes, thinly sliced

1 yellow or white onion, thinly sliced

2 tablespoons finely chopped fresh parsley

¼ teaspoon freshly ground black pepper

¼ cup Vegetable Broth (page 59)

1. Spray a medium-sized skillet with nonstick cooking spray. Alternate slices of potatoes and onions in a winding circle around the pan. Sprinkle with parsley and black pepper, add the broth, and bring to a boil. Reduce the heat to low, cover, and cook for 30 minutes, or until the potatoes are tender and the liquid has been absorbed.

2. Serve immediately.

TAKE A CHANCE:

• Instead of a skillet, arrange the potato and onion slices in an ovenproof casserole dish. Sauté 1 clove of minced garlic in 3 tablespoons soy margarine, then drizzle it over the potatoes. Cover the dish and bake in a 400°F oven for 25 minutes, or until the potatoes are cooked. Uncover and bake another 10 minutes to brown the potatoes.

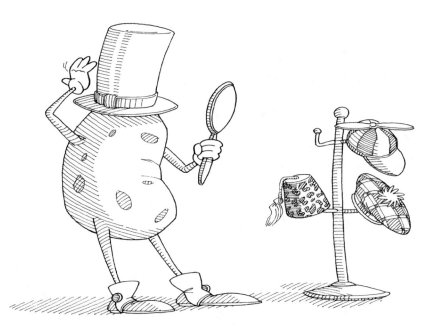

Potato & Onion Cake Wales

YIELD: 4 SERVINGS   PREPARATION TIME: 1¾ HOURS

1. Melt the margarine in a small saucepan over low heat. Add the black pepper and stir. Remove from the heat and set aside.

2. Spray a round ovenproof casserole dish with nonstick cooking spray. Place a layer of potatoes in the bottom of the dish and top with a layer of onions. Spoon a tablespoon of the melted margarine over the onions. Continue the layering, making sure to top with a layer of potatoes. Pour any remaining margarine on top.

3. Cover and bake in a 300°F oven for 1 hour. Uncover and bake another 30 minutes.

4. Remove the dish from the oven, let it stand for a minute or two, then invert it on an ovenproof plate. Remove the dish and place the "cake" under the broiler for 2 to 3 minutes, or until the potatoes begin to brown.

5. Garnish with chives, cut into wedges, and serve.

TAKE A CHANCE:

• Reduce the margarine to 2 tablespoons and add 2 to 3 tablespoons Vegetable Broth (page 59).

• Add slices of green pepper between the layers.

This very old Welsh recipe is similar to the Stovies (page 132) from Scotland. In this dish, the potatoes are slowly baked in the oven.

¼ cup soy margarine

¼ teaspoon freshly ground black pepper

4 baking potatoes, thinly sliced

3 onions, coarsely chopped

2 tablespoons chopped chives

Creamy Potatoes & Onions Sweden

We've deviated from the original Swedish recipe by substituting whipped tofu for the cream. These potatoes are like creamy home fries.

4 ounces firm tofu, drained

1/2 cup skim milk

2 tablespoons canola oil

2 onions, coarsely chopped

4 large baking potatoes, diced

1/2 teaspoon freshly ground black pepper

2 teaspoons finely chopped fresh parsley

YIELD: 4 SERVINGS   PREPARATION TIME: 45 MINUTES

1. Place the tofu in a food processor and pulse three times. Add the milk and blend the mixture until it is smooth. Set aside.

2. Melt the margarine in a large skillet over medium heat. Add the onions and sauté for 5 minutes. Reduce the heat to medium-low, add the potatoes, and cook covered for 20 minutes, or until they are browned. Sprinkle with black pepper.

3. Slowly add the tofu mixture to the skillet, and stir to coat the potatoes. Gently simmer uncovered for 15 minutes, or until the potatoes are tender.

4. Garnish with parsley and serve immediately.

TAKE A CHANCE:

• Thinly slice the potatoes and onions instead of dicing and chopping them.

• Use a combination of onions, shallots, and leeks, instead of all onions.

• Garnish with chopped garlic chives instead of parsley.

• Use Creamy Roasted Garlic Sauce (page 169) instead of plain tofu.

Roasted Vidalias United States

YIELD: 4 SERVINGS   PREPARATION TIME: 1 HOUR

1. In a small bowl, mix together the vinegar, olive oil, and black pepper.

2. Place the onions on a large square of foil. Bring up the sides of the foil, add the liquid, and seal the foil tightly into a packet.

3. Set the packet on a baking sheet and place in a 350°F oven. Bake for 50 to 60 minutes, or until the onions are tender.

4. Transfer the roasted onions to a serving bowl and enjoy as an accompaniment to just about any meal.

TAKE A CHANCE:

• Cook the onions in an onion roaster. Pour the vinegar, olive oil, and black pepper on top of the onions. Cover the roaster and bake the onions in a 350°F oven for 50 to 60 minutes, or until they are tender.

• Use $1/2$ cup Vegetable Broth (page 59) instead of the olive oil and vinegar.

• Top the onions with a dollop of Pesto Sauce (page 172) before serving.

Vidalias are the most popular variety of specialty sweet onions grown in the United States. Roasting makes this sweet onion even sweeter.

$1/4$ cup balsamic vinegar

2 tablespoons extra-virgin olive oil

$1/4$ teaspoon freshly ground black pepper

4 Vidalia onions, peeled and left whole

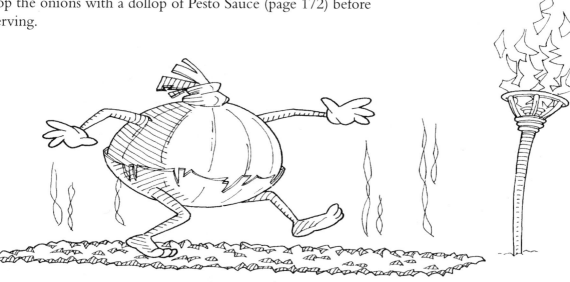

Broiled Onions with Raisin Sauce United States

This slightly sweet raisin sauce tempers any remaining heat in the broiled onions. Serve as an accompaniment to Onion Leek Risotto (page 98).

4 yellow or white onions

1 teaspoon safflower oil

1/4 cup water

1/4 cup fruit-juice concentrate (juice blend)

2 tablespoons soy margarine

1 tablespoon arrowroot

1/4 cup dark raisins

YIELD: 4 SERVINGS   PREPARATION TIME: 10 MINUTES

1. Being careful not to cut them all the way through, quarter the onions to within an inch of their bottoms. Place them on a broiler pan and drizzle with oil. Broil the onions for 10 minutes, or until they are cooked through.

2. Place the water, fruit-juice concentrate, and margarine in a small saucepan over medium-high heat. When the margarine melts, add the arrowroot and stir constantly for 5 minutes, or until the sauce begins to thicken. Reduce the heat to medium-low, add the raisins, and cook for 5 minutes.

3. Place the broiled onions on a serving dish and spoon the sauce on top. Serve immediately.

TAKE A CHANCE:

- Stir 2 tablespoons chopped walnuts or almonds into the sauce before serving.

- Use golden raisins instead of dark.

Trivia Tidbit

The more pungent a raw onion is, the sweeter it becomes after cooking.

Fresh Peas with Pearl Onions France

YIELD: 4 SERVINGS PREPARATION TIME: 10 MINUTES

1. Bring the peas, onions, and water to a boil in a medium saucepan. Cook over medium heat for 5 minutes. Drain.

2. Serve immediately.

TAKE A CHANCE:

• Use frozen peas.

• Use 1 or 2 chopped shallots instead of pearl onions.

• Add 10 finely chopped mint leaves to the peas before serving.

Pearl onions are small, flavorful nuggets. When added to fresh green peas, they help to create a delicious side dish for any meal.

2 cups fresh green peas

8 pearl onions, skin removed

1/2 cup water

Sweet Glazed Pearl Onions Finland

YIELD: 4 SERVINGS PREPARATION TIME: 25 MINUTES

1. Bring a large saucepan of water to a boil. Add the onions and blanch for 5 minutes. Drain, cool, and remove the skins.

2. Melt the margarine in a large skillet over medium heat. Add the molasses, broth, and soy sauce, and cook for 1 minute. Stir in the rosemary and mustard, and mix well.

3. Reduce the heat to low. Add the onions and cook for 10 to 12 minutes, or until the onions are golden brown and well-covered with the glaze.

4. Serve immediately.

TAKE A CHANCE:

• Use boiling onions instead of pearl onions.

• Use honey instead of molasses.

Sweetened with a touch of molasses, these small onions are an excellent addition to any meal. Be sure to try them with Spicy Chicken Fajitas (page 104).

1 pound pearl onions, unpeeled

1 tablespoon soy margarine

1 tablespoon molasses

2 teaspoons Vegetable Broth (page 59)

1 teaspoon shoyu or tamari soy sauce

1/2 teaspoon dried rosemary

1 teaspoon dried mustard

Braised Red Cabbage Germany

Germans use lots of onions in their cooking. This recipe combines onions with tart apples and mellow cabbage. Keep in mind that the red cabbage will lose its bright color when cooked.

1/4 cup Vegetable Broth (page 59)

1 yellow or white onion, finely chopped

5 cups finely shredded red cabbage

3 tart apples, cored, pared, and thinly sliced

1/2 cup water

3 whole cloves

1 bay leaf

2 tablespoons date sugar

2 tablespoons red wine vinegar

1 teaspoon arrowroot

YIELD: 4 SERVINGS   PREPARATION TIME: 45 MINUTES

1. Place the broth in a large skillet over medium heat. Add the onion and sauté for 2 minutes, then toss in the cabbage and sauté an additional 5 minutes. Reduce the heat to low and add all of the remaining ingredients, except the arrowroot. Cover and cook for approximately 15 minutes, or until the cabbage is tender.

2. Remove 1/4 cup of liquid from the skillet and place it in a small bowl. Add the arrowroot and mix well. Slowly return the mixture to the skillet. Stirring occasionally, continue to cook 5 minutes, or until the liquid thickens.

3. Serve immediately.

TAKE A CHANCE:

• Use green cabbage instead of red.

• Add 1 teaspoon caraway seeds.

Trivia Tidbit

Does your garden seem to be a popular dining spot for pesky rabbits? Planting onions, garlic, or leeks in a border around your vegetables should help to keep them out.

Sauerkraut Germany

YIELD: 4 SERVINGS   PREPARATION TIME: 45 MINUTES

1. Place the oil in a large saucepan over medium heat. Add the onions and sauté for 10 minutes, then add the sauerkraut and continue to sauté another 5 minutes. Add the water, mix well, and reduce the heat to medium-low. Cover and cook for 25 minutes.

2. Add the potato and continue to cook for 10 minutes. Stir in the sugar and black pepper. Mix well.

3. Serve immediately.

TAKE A CHANCE:

• Halfway through the sauerkraut's cooking time, add 1 cup peeled and chopped apples. Taste the sauerkraut before adding the sugar. It may not be needed.

• For a Hungarian version, omit the potato and add 1 teaspoon sweet Hungarian paprika and $^1/_2$ teaspoon caraway seeds.

This traditional German dish combines onions with tart sauerkraut for a tasty treat.

2 teaspoons canola oil

2 yellow or white onions, thinly sliced

4 cups sauerkraut, unwashed

1 cup water

1 potato, peeled and grated

$^1/_2$ teaspoon date sugar

$^1/_4$ teaspoon freshly ground black pepper

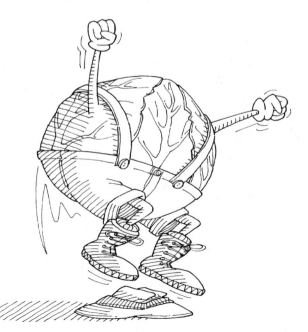

Baked Sauerkraut Russia

This dish takes a while to bake, but the result is sauerkraut with a very mellow taste. Serve as a side dish or a main meal.

4 cups sauerkraut, rinsed well and drained

4 cups thinly sliced green cabbage

2 tablespoons canola oil

4 onions, thinly sliced

1 cup water

$1/4$ teaspoon freshly ground black pepper

YIELD: 6 SERVINGS   PREPARATION TIME: $2^1/2$ HOURS

1. Mix the sauerkraut and cabbage together in a 3-quart oven-proof casserole dish.

2. Place the oil in a skillet over medium heat. Add the onions and sauté for 15 minutes. Transfer the onions to the casserole dish along with the water and black pepper. Mix well.

3. Place in a 350°F oven and bake covered for $1^1/2$ hours. Uncover and bake another 30 minutes. Add a little more water if needed to keep the casserole from drying out.

4. Serve immediately with Beet Salad (page 48) and Onion Flat Bread (page 181).

TAKE A CHANCE:

• Use $1/2$ cup water and $1/2$ cup Vegetable Broth (page 59) instead of all water.

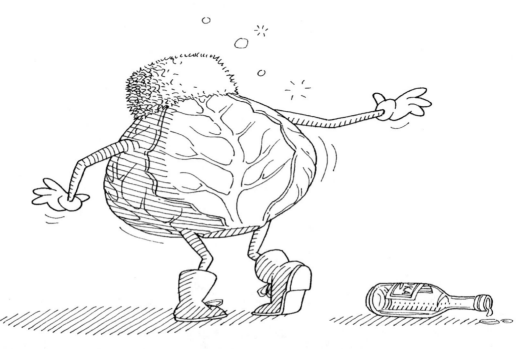

Cabbage & Onions India

YIELD: 4 SERVINGS   PREPARATION TIME: 1 HOUR

1. Place 2 tablespoons of the oil in a large skillet over medium heat. Add the fenugreek, mustard seeds, fennel seeds, and cumin seeds, and cook for 1 minute, or until the seeds start to change colors. Add $1^1/2$ of the chopped onions and sauté for 5 minutes. Reduce the heat to medium-low, add the cabbage, and cook for 30 minutes.

2. Blend the garlic and tomato in a food processor until smooth. Add the ginger and continue to blend until a paste is formed.

3. Heat the remaining oil in a small skillet, and add the tomato paste, chili peppers, and turmeric. Simmer for 5 minutes, then add to the cabbage along with the garam masala and lemon juice. Stir well and continue to cook an additional 5 minutes.

4. Place in a serving bowl and enjoy immediately.

TAKE A CHANCE:

• Reduce the amount of onions to 1 and add 4 large chopped shallots.

Onions are an important ingredient in Indian cooking. Here they are added to cabbage and simmered in aromatic spices.

4 tablespoons canola oil

4 whole fenugreek seeds, or $1/8$ teaspoon ground fenugreek

$1/2$ teaspoon mustard seeds

$1/2$ teaspoon fennel seeds

$1/2$ teaspoon cumin seeds

2 onions, coarsely chopped

4 cups finely shredded cabbage

3 cloves garlic, finely chopped

1 small tomato, coarsely chopped

2 teaspoons freshly grated ginger

2 serrano chili peppers, seeded and finely chopped

$1/2$ teaspoon ground turmeric

$1/2$ teaspoon garam masala*

2 tablespoons fresh lemon juice

* This combination of spices used in Indian cuisine is available in gourmet shops, specialty shops, and some grocery stores.

Baked Honey Onions Croatia

Another sweetened onion dish, this time covered in cheese.

1 cup Chicken Broth (page 58)

1 tablespoon soy margarine, melted

2 teaspoons honey

1/4 teaspoon lemon rind

1/4 teaspoon paprika

1/4 teaspoon freshly ground black pepper

2 tablespoons finely chopped fresh parsley

3 large white onions, quartered

1 cup shredded lowfat cheddar cheese

YIELD: 4 SERVINGS   PREPARATION TIME: 1 1/4 HOURS

1. Mix all of the ingredients, except the onions and cheese, together in a bowl.

2. Coat a 2-quart ovenproof casserole dish with nonstick cooking spray. Arrange the onions in a single layer in the dish and cover with the liquid.

3. Bake covered in a 325°F oven for 1 hour. Uncover and sprinkle the cheese on top. Return to the oven and bake for 5 minutes, or until the cheese is melted.

4. Serve hot.

TAKE A CHANCE:

• Reduce the number of onions to 2, and add the white part of 2 or 3 leeks that have been halved.

Scalloped Onions Croatia

YIELD: 4 SERVINGS PREPARATION TIME: 45 MINUTES

1. Melt the margarine in a medium saucepan over medium heat. Stir in the flour, and blend until smooth. Slowly add the broth, stirring constantly to prevent lumps from forming. Add the black pepper and cook, stirring constantly, until the sauce is thick and starts to bubble.

2. Coat a 1½-quart ovenproof casserole dish with nonstick cooking spray. Arrange the onions in the dish and cover with the liquid. Sprinkle the cheese and walnuts on top. Cover and bake in a 375°F oven for 30 minutes.

3. Serve hot.

TAKE A CHANCE:

• Add ¼ teaspoon cayenne pepper to the sauce.

• Use almonds instead of walnuts.

We love the crunchy texture of the onions in this Croatian classic.

3 tablespoons soy margarine

3 tablespoons unbleached white flour

1½ cups Chicken Broth (page 58)

⅛ teaspoon freshly ground black pepper

3 large white onions, thinly sliced

½ cup shredded nonfat cheddar cheese

½ cup coarsely chopped walnuts

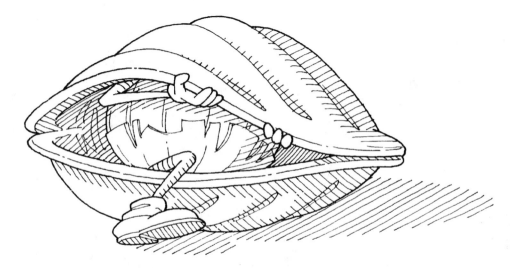

Spicy Steamed Vegetables *Ethiopia*

These are not your ordinary tasteless steamed vegetables. Tossed with a spicy mixture of onions and garlic, these vegetables will add zip to any meal.

4 new or red potatoes, quartered

2 large carrots, peeled and cut into $1/4$-inch slices

1 green bell pepper, seeded and cut into $1/2$-inch pieces

4 ounces green beans, trimmed

2 tablespoons soy margarine

$1/2$ teaspoon turmeric

2 onions, finely chopped

3 cloves garlic, finely chopped

2 tablespoons Berbere Sauce (page 166)

1 teaspoon freshly grated ginger

2 tablespoons fresh lemon juice

YIELD: 4 SERVINGS   PREPARATION TIME: 25 MINUTES

1. Cook the potatoes on a vegetable steamer for 3 minutes. Add the carrots, bell pepper, and beans, and steam for 5 minutes or until the vegetables are tender yet crisp. (Do not overcook.)

2. Melt the margarine in a small saucepan over medium heat. Add the onions and sauté for 5 minutes. Add the garlic, Berbere Sauce, and ginger, and cook another minute. Remove the pan from the heat and stir in the lemon juice.

3. Place the vegetables in a large serving bowl and toss with the sauce.

TAKE A CHANCE:

• Add 3 seeded and chopped jalapeño chili peppers to the sauce.

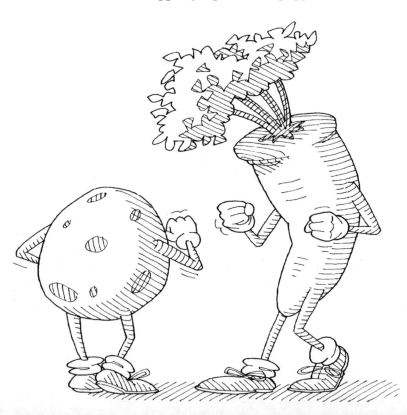

Black Beans Cuba / Latin America / American Southwest

YIELD: 4 SERVINGS PREPARATION TIME: 20 MINUTES

1. Place the broth in a large skillet over medium heat. Add the onions and sauté for 5 minutes, then add the garlic and sauté another minute.

2. Toss in the bell peppers, chili peppers, and tomatoes, and continue to sauté for 5 minutes. Stir in the black beans, oregano, cayenne pepper, and black pepper, and cook for 1 minute.

3. Spoon the beans into a serving bowl and top with the cheese, cilantro, and scallions.

TAKE A CHANCE:

• Omit the bell peppers, chili peppers, and tomatoes, and increase the broth to $1/2$ cup. Garnish as desired.

Trivia Tidbit

Onions and garlic are so ingrained in South American cookery, that they are used in many traditional South American Indian dishes.

Black beans are hot items, and not just in taste. They are showing up in soups and salads, and as side dishes. Serve these at your next barbecue instead of baked beans.

$1/4$ cup Vegetable Broth (page 59)

2 yellow and white onions, finely chopped

4 cloves garlic, finely chopped

2 green bell peppers, seeded and cut into $1/2$-inch pieces

1 red bell pepper, seeded and cut into $1/2$-inch pieces

2 poblano chili peppers, seeded and chopped

2 jalapeño chili peppers, seeded and chopped

3 large tomatoes, seeded and chopped

2 cups cooked black beans

1 teaspoon oregano

$1/4$ teaspoon cayenne pepper

$1/4$ teaspoon freshly ground black pepper

$1/4$ cup shredded Monterey Jack cheese

$1/4$ cup finely chopped fresh cilantro

4 scallions, coarsely chopped

Onion Tart Switzerland

This may seem like a lot of onions to slice, but they will cook down to just the right amount in this tasty tart. Serve as a side dish or as an appetizer with a different twist.

Crust

1 cup whole wheat pastry flour

1/4 cup canola oil

3 tablespoons hot water

Filling

2 teaspoons soy margarine

8 cups onions, thinly sliced

1/2 cup egg substitute, or 2 eggs

1 cup skim milk

1/4 teaspoon freshly ground black pepper

YIELD: 8- OR 9-INCH TART   PREPARATION TIME: 1 HOUR

1. To make the crust, place the flour in a large bowl and stir in the oil. The mixture should resemble cornmeal. Sprinkle the flour mixture with just enough hot water, 2 tablespoons at a time, to form a dough that almost cleans the sides of the bowl. Add 1 to 2 more teaspoons of water, if necessary.

2. Shape the dough into a ball and flatten it on a lightly floured work surface. Using a floured rolling pin, roll the dough into a circle that is 2 inches larger than the tart pan.

3. Place the dough in the tart pan and gently press it against the bottom and sides. Trim away the overhanging dough. Using a fork, prick the dough on the bottom and sides.

4. Bake the crust in a 475°F oven for 5 minutes. Set aside.

5. To make the filling, melt the margarine in a large skillet over medium heat. Add the onions and sauté for 10 minutes, then place them in the pie crust.

6. In a small bowl, beat together the eggs and milk, then pour it over the onions.

7. Bake the tart in a 350°F for 20 minutes, or until set.

8. Remove from the oven, cut into slices, and serve.

TAKE A CHANCE:

• Add 1/4 cup crumbled turkey bacon to the onions.

• Reduce the onions by 1 or 2 cups, and add a like amount of thinly sliced leeks.

Grated Cheese & Onion Pie England

*T*his tasty double-crust pie is almost a meal in itself.

1. To make the crust, place the flour in a large bowl and stir in the oil. The mixture should resemble cornmeal. Sprinkle the flour mixture with just enough hot water, 1 tablespoon at a time, to form a dough that almost cleans the sides of the bowl. Add 1 to 2 more teaspoons of water, if necessary.

2. Divide the dough in half and shape each half into a ball. Place the balls on a lightly floured work surface. Using a floured rolling pin, roll each ball of dough into a 10-inch circle.

3. Place one of the circles in the pie pan and gently press it against the bottom and sides, allowing the dough to extend $1/4$ inch over the edge. Trim away any excess dough. Place the onions and cheese on top of the crust, and set aside.

4. Place the tofu, 3 tablespoons of the milk, the nutmeg, and the black pepper in a food processor and blend for 1 minute, or until the mixture is smooth and creamy. Pour the mixture over the onions and cheese.

5. Drape the remaining circle of dough over the filled crust. Press the edges of the top and bottom crusts together, then roll up the edges and crimp. Brush the remaining milk over the top crust.

6. Bake the pie in a 350°F oven for 40 to 45 minutes, or until the top is golden brown.

7. Remove the pie from the oven, slice, and serve.

Crust

2 cups whole wheat pastry flour

$1/2$ cup canola oil

6 tablespoons hot water

Filling

2 yellow or white onions, grated

1 cup grated sharp cheddar cheese

8 ounces firm silken tofu, drained

4 tablespoons skim milk

$1/4$ teaspoon nutmeg

$1/4$ teaspoon freshly ground black pepper

TAKE A CHANCE:

• Make individual tarts with single or double crusts.

Vegetable Kebabs Turkey

A variation on shish kebab, these vegetables are saturated in a garlic marinade before grilling.

1 yellow or white onion, halved lengthwise, then cut into 1-inch slices

12 cherry tomatoes

12 large mushrooms, stems removed

1 large zucchini, cut into 1-inch slices

1 large crookneck squash, cut into 1-inch pieces

1 large green pepper, seeded and cut into 1-inch squares

Marinade

6 cloves garlic, crushed

3 tablespoons fresh lemon juice

2 tablespoons extra-virgin olive oil

$^1/_2$ teaspoon oregano

YIELD: 4 SERVINGS   PREPARATION TIME: 1$^1/_2$ HOURS

1. Combine the marinade ingredients in a large bowl. Add the vegetables, mix well, and refrigerate for 1 hour.

2. Alternate threading the marinated vegetables on metal skewers (or bamboo skewers that have been soaked in water for 30 minutes).

3. Turning and basting them frequently with the marinade, grill the kebabs on the barbecue for 15 minutes, or until the vegetables are tender.

4. Serve immediately over Baked Rice (page 99).

TAKE A CHANCE:

• Use 12 pearl onions instead of onion slices.

• Add 4 leeks, white part only, cut into quarters.

• Omit the marinade and baste the vegetables in Pesto Sauce (page 172) as they cook.

Stewed Onions, Eggplant, & Tomatoes Israel

YIELD: 4 SERVINGS   PREPARATION TIME: 30 MINUTES

1. Place the broth in a large skillet over medium heat. Add the onions and sauté for 5 minutes, then add the garlic and sauté another minute. Stir in the eggplant, tomatoes, turmeric, and black pepper, and cook for 15 minutes, or until the vegetables are tender. Stir in the lemon juice.

2. Transfer the vegetables to a serving bowl, garnish with cilantro, and serve immediately.

TAKE A CHANCE:

• Add 2 seeded and finely chopped jalapeño chili peppers, or 1 teaspoon crushed red pepper.

• Add 3 tablespoons tomato sauce.

This slow-simmered, savory vegetable combination is an easy-to-make side dish. You can also tuck it into a pita pocket or use it as a topping for baked potatoes or pasta.

1/4 cup Vegetable Broth (page 59)

2 yellow or white onions, thinly sliced

4 cloves garlic, finely chopped

1 eggplant, peeled and cut into 1-inch cubes

3 tomatoes, chopped

1/2 teaspoon turmeric

1/4 teaspoon freshly ground black pepper

1/4 cup fresh lemon juice

2 teaspoons finely chopped cilantro

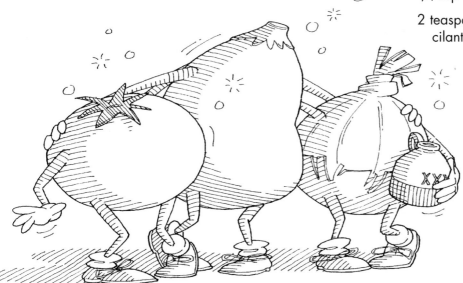

Onions & Peppers Italy / United States

This is another great topping for baked potatoes. You can also try mixing it with Garlic Mashed Potatoes (page 127).

1/4 cup Vegetable Broth (page 59)

3 tablespoons soy margarine

2 yellow or white onions, halved lengthwise then cut into 1/4-inch slices

3 green bell peppers, seeded and cut into 1/4-inch slices

1/4 teaspoon freshly ground black pepper

YIELD: 4 SERVINGS   PREPARATION TIME: 40 MINUTES

1. Place the broth in a large skillet over medium heat. Add the onions and sauté for 10 minutes. Reduce the heat to low, and add the bell peppers and black pepper. Cover and cook for 20 minutes, stirring occasionally. Add additional broth if necessary.

2. Serve immediately.

TAKE A CHANCE:

• Use only 1 onion and add 4 thinly sliced leeks, white part only, or 6 thinly sliced shallots.

• For added color, use a combination of green, red, and yellow bell peppers.

Yucca in Garlic Sauce Cuba

YIELD: 4 SERVINGS   PREPARATION TIME: 45 MINUTES

1. Place the yucca in a large saucepan, cover with water, and bring to a boil. Reduce the heat to medium–low, cover, and cook the yucca for 30 minutes, or until it is tender.

2. Combine the lemon juice and oil in a small saucepan over medium heat. Add the garlic and sauté for 1 minute.

3. Transfer the cooked yucca to a serving bowl, add the garlic sauce, and toss to coat. Serve immediately.

TAKE A CHANCE:

• Use white potatoes or sweet potatoes instead of yucca.

• Mash the yucca before mixing it with the sauce.

Yucca (cassava) is a root vegetable and a staple in Cuban cooking. Its taste is similar but more delicate than a sweet potato. You can find yucca in Hispanic markets, gourmet shops, and some grocery stores.

2 pounds yucca, peeled and cut into $1/2$-inch cubes

$1/2$ cup fresh lemon juice

3 tablespoons extra-virgin olive oil

6 cloves garlic, crushed

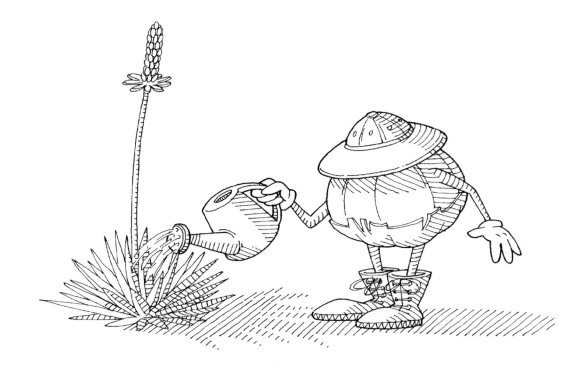

Chapter 8

Pungent Accompaniments

There is no reason any meal should go it alone. You can add garlic and onion accompaniments to bring excitement and passion to any meal. The easy-to-make allium-based sauces, dressings, and tidbits presented in this chapter are guaranteed to deliver enough gusto to turn ordinary fare into a festival of flavors.

Crispy Onions Indonesia / India

Slowly browned to perfection, these onions are a wonderful garnish for vegetables, rice, and noodles. Try some with Cabbage & Onions (page 141) or Baked Rice (page 99).

1 yellow or white onion, thinly sliced

1/2 cup safflower oil

YIELD: 3/4 CUP   PREPARATION TIME: 10 MINUTES

1. Spread the onion slices on paper toweling to dry.

2. Place the oil in a skillet or wok over medium-high heat. Add the onions and cook for 5 minutes, stirring constantly. Reduce the heat to medium and cook another 5 minutes, or until the onions are crisp and golden brown. With a slotted spoon, remove the onions to a dish lined with paper toweling.

3. Serve immediately.

TAKE A CHANCE:

• Following the same instructions, make Crispy Garlic slices. Be careful not to let the garlic brown too much or too quickly. This can cause it to burn and become bitter.

Trivia Tidbit

Although it takes only a minute for sautéed garlic to go from browned to burnt, there is a big difference between the two. Browned garlic has a wonderful earthy taste and aroma, while burnt garlic is acrid and bitter, and must be discarded. Always keep an eye on garlic as it browns, and follow your nose. When you smell its strong aroma, the garlic is done.

Pickled Onions England

YIELD: 1 QUART   PREPARATION TIME: 2 WEEKS

1. Bring a large saucepan of water to a boil. Add the onions and boil them for 1 minute, then remove and drain. When the onions are cool enough to handle, peel away their skin, rub them with salt, and place them in a large bowl, Cover and refrigerate overnight.

2. Rinse the onions and pat dry with paper toweling.

3. Place the vinegar, peppercorns, cloves, and sugar in a large saucepan over medium heat, and simmer 2 minutes, or until the sugar is dissolved. Add the onions. if necessary, add more water to completely cover the onions. Bring the ingredients to a boil, then reduce the heat to medium–low, Simmer the onions for 10 minutes, or until they are soft on the outside but hard and crunchy on the inside.

4. Using a slotted spoon, transfer the onions to a sterilized quart jar and cover with the vinegar mixture. Seal tightly and store in the refrigerator for 2 weeks before using.

TAKE A CHANCE:

• Add a whole small mushrooms to the jar along with the onions.

• Use malt vinegar instead of white.

These tart beauties can enjoyed alone or as a side dish. Try them with Shepherd's Pie (page 91).

12 small boiling onions

1/2 cup sea salt

3 cups distilled white vinegar

10 whole peppercorns, black or mixed colors

6 whole cloves

6 tablespoons date sugar

Trivia Tidbit

While onions are common ingredients in the cuisine of England, garlic is rarely used.

Pickled Onion Rings Croatia

These crunchy onion rings need only three days to marinate. Serve as an accompaniment to Spicy Orange & Onion Salad (page 52).

2 large yellow or white onions, cut into $1/2$-inch slices

2 cups commercial pickle juice

YIELD: APPROXIMATELY 1 QUART   PREPARATION TIME: 3 DAYS

1. Separate the onion slices into individual rings. Place the rings in a quart-sized glass jar and completely cover with pickle juice.

2. Seal tightly and refrigerate for 3 days before serving.

TAKE A CHANCE:

• Add 2 or 3 whole garlic cloves to the jar.

Hot Pickled Onions India

Similar to the English version on page 155, these onions have a bit more kick. Serve them with Baked Rice (page 99).

10 small boiling onions

3 cloves garlic, thinly sliced

3 dried serrano or Thai chili peppers

2 cups red wine vinegar

YIELD: 1 QUART   PREPARATION TIME: 1$1/2$ DAYS

1. Bring a large saucepan of water to a boil. Add the onions and boil them for 1 minute, then remove and drain. When the onions are cool enough to handle, peel away their skin.

2. Being careful not to cut them all the way through, quarter each onion to within a $1/2$-inch of their bottoms. Place the onions, cut side up, in a sterilized quart jar. Add the remaining ingredients, seal tightly, and let sit at least 1 day before using.

3. Once the jar has been opened, store it in the refrigerator. The onions will keep for about 3 weeks.

TAKE A CHANCE:

• Add 12 whole peppercorns (black or mixed colors) to the jar.

Lime-Marinated Onion Rings Mexico

YIELD: 2 CUPS   PREPARATION TIME: 2 HOURS

1. Separate the onions into individual rings and place in a glass bowl or jar. Add the lime juice and salt and mix well.

2. Cover and refrigerate for at least 2 hours before serving.

TAKE A CHANCE:

• Use half lime and half lemon juice.

• Add some small dried chili peppers, or 1 teaspoon crushed red pepper flakes.

• Use a sweet onion such as Vidalia or Spanish instead of the red.

These marinated onions are the easiest you can make, and the flavor of lime will transport you South of the Border. Use these onions to top the Antipasto on page 44.

2 cups red onions, thinly sliced

$1/4$ cup fresh lime juice

$1/2$ teaspoon sea salt

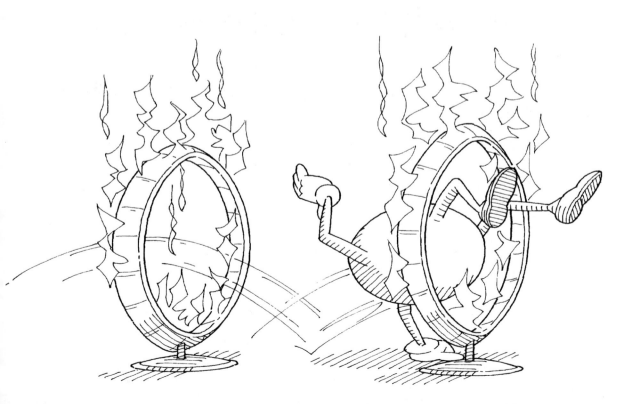

Pickled Garlic Thailand

Pickling garlic allows Thai cooks to keep this indispensable ingredient almost indefinitely. Be warned, chomping down on this pickled garlic is an acquired taste. Serve alongside Crispy Noodles with Garlic & Shallots (page 101).

1 1/2 cups white vinegar

1 teaspoon date sugar

40 cloves garlic (about 4 heads), peeled

YIELD: 3 CUPS   PREPARATION TIME: 1 WEEK

1. Place the vinegar and sugar in a small saucepan over medium heat for 10 minutes, or until the sugar is dissolved. Cool.

2. Put the garlic cloves in a quart-sized sterilized glass jar, add the vinegar, and seal. Refrigerate for 1 week before serving.

TAKE A CHANCE:

• Add 1 or 2 dried chili peppers to the jar for a spark of heat.

• The garlic cloves can be added to the jar with their skin on. Just peel before using.

Garlic Croutons France

These crunchy croutons have a lively garlic taste that will wake up any salad.

4 cloves garlic, crushed

3 slices stale French bread, cut into 1/2-inch cubes

3 tablespoons soy margarine

YIELD: 1 CUP   PREPARATION TIME: 30 MINUTES

1. Place the bread cubes on a cookie sheet, and bake in a 250°F oven for 15 minutes, or until the cubes are completely dry and lightly browned.

2. Melt the margarine in a large skillet over medium heat. Add the garlic and sauté lightly for 1 minute. Add the bread cubes to the skillet and stir gently until they have absorbed the margarine.

3. Cool the croutons before using in soups and salads.

TAKE A CHANCE:

• Use whole wheat or multi-grain bread.

• Use pita bread that has been cut into 2-inch triangles.

Garlic Lemon Vinaigrette Greece

YIELD: ½ CUP   PREPARATION TIME: 30 MINUTES

1. Combine all of the ingredients in a glass jar or bottle and shake until well-blended. Let stand for 20 minutes.
2. Pour the desired amount over salad and toss.
3. Tightly cover the remaining dressing and refrigerate up to 2 days.

TAKE A CHANCE:

• Use finely chopped fresh mint instead of oregano.

• Try this vinaigrette over warm pasta for a refreshing side dish.

Our two favorite ingredients—garlic and lemon—are combined for a refreshing taste that can be used on any salad.

3 cloves garlic, finely chopped

¼ cup extra-virgin olive oil

1 teaspoon dried oregano

¼ teaspoon freshly ground black pepper

Balsamic Vinaigrette with Garlic & Shallots France

YIELD: ½ CUP   PREPARATION TIME: 10 MINUTES

1. Place all of the ingredients in a glass jar or bottle and shake well.
2. Pour the desired amount over salad and toss.
3. Tightly cover the remaining dressing and refrigerate up to 2 days.

TAKE A CHANCE:

• Reduce the vinegar or the olive oil, and add an equal amount of lemon juice.

Made with two essential French ingredients—garlic and shallots—this rich vinaigrette is great over spinach salad.

¼ cup balsamic vinegar

¼ cup extra-virgin olive oil

2 large shallots, thinly sliced

1 clove garlic, thinly sliced

1 tablespoon finely chopped fresh parsley

Garlic Shoyu Dip Philippines

Serve this as an accompaniment to grilled tofu, chicken, or fish, or use it as a marinade.

4 cloves garlic, crushed

1/4 cup shoyu or tamari sauce

1/3 cup distilled white vinegar

1/2 teaspoon crushed red pepper

YIELD: 3/4 CUP   PREPARATION TIME: 30 MINUTES

1. Place all of the ingredients in a glass jar or bottle and shake well.
2. Refrigerate for 30 minutes. Shake well before using.

TAKE A CHANCE:

- Use 2 small dried red peppers instead of crushed pepper.
- Use a reduced-sodium shoyu or tamari sauce.

Red Onion Vinaigrette Austria

Tart with wine vinegar and mustard, this vinaigrette is great on a salad of curly endive. We also use it as a marinade for broiled chicken.

1/4 cup extra-virgin olive oil

1/4 cup red or white wine vinegar

1 red onion, coarsely chopped

2 cloves garlic, finely chopped

2 tablespoons finely chopped fresh chives

2 tablespoons finely chopped fresh parsley

4 teaspoons prepared mustard (preferably Dijon-style)

YIELD: 1 1/4 CUPS   PREPARATION TIME: 10 MINUTES

1. Place all of the ingredients in a small bowl and mix well.
2. Cover and refrigerate for 30 minutes before using.

TAKE A CHANCE:

- To use as a marinade for broiled chicken, reduce the vinegar to 2 tablespoons. The marinade can be used immediately.

Piquant Tomato Sauce Mexico

YIELD: 2 CUPS   PREPARATION TIME: 25 MINUTES

1. Place the oil in a large skillet over medium heat. Add the oregano and sauté for 1 minute, then toss in the onion, garlic, and chili peppers, and continue to sauté for 5 minutes. Add the tomatoes and continue to cook for 15 minutes, stirring often.

2. Serve hot or warm.

TAKE A CHANCE:

• Roast the jalapeño peppers for a smoky taste.

• Use 6 cloves Roasted Garlic (page 25) instead of the fresh.

• Place all of the cooked ingredients in a food processor and blend until smooth. Return the sauce to the pan and heat again before serving.

This sauce can be used as an accompaniment for a wide range of dishes—from tofu and eggs to chicken and fish. We like it as a topping for baked potatoes, as well as a sauce for simple roasted chicken.

2 tablespoons canola oil

1 teaspoon finely chopped fresh oregano

1 yellow or white onion, finely chopped

4 cloves garlic, finely chopped

4 jalapeño chili peppers, seeded and finely chopped

5 large tomatoes, coarsely chopped

Trivia Tidbit

If onions upset your stomach, use shallots, which are easier on the digestive system. Shallots are also milder than onions in both flavor and aroma.

Backyard Barbecue Sauce United States

Try this zesty barbecue sauce on any grilled food—we love it on tofu burgers. Just make sure there is enough to go around.

1 1/2 cups ketchup

1/4 cup fresh lemon juice

2 cloves garlic, thinly sliced lengthwise

1/2-inch thick slice of yellow or white onion

1 teaspoon cayenne pepper

1 teaspoon shoyu or tamari soy sauce

1/2 teaspoon dried thyme

1/2 teaspoon dried sage

1/4 teaspoon freshly ground black pepper

YIELD: 1 3/4 CUPS   PREPARATION TIME: 1 1/2 HOURS

1. Mix all of the ingredients in a bowl. Cover and let sit at room temperature for 1 hour.

2. Discard the onion slice and brush the sauce on grilled foods near the end of their cooking time. Serve the remaining sauce on the side.

TAKE A CHANCE:

• Use Worcestershire instead of soy sauce.

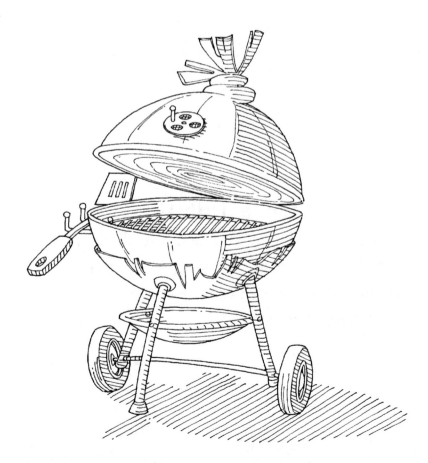

Onion Sauce Germany

YIELD: 2 CUPS   PREPARATION TIME: 20 MINUTES

1. Place $1/4$ cup of the broth in a large skillet over medium heat. Add the onions and sauté for 20 minutes. Slowly stir in the arrowroot until it is completely dissolved. Add the remaining broth and the caraway seeds. Bring the ingredients to a boil, then reduce the heat to medium-low and simmer for 10 minutes.

2. Pour the sauce through a wire mesh strainer that is set over a medium saucepan. Using the back of a spoon, press the solids through the strainer and back into the liquid.

3. Place the saucepan over medium heat. Add the vinegar and sugar, and cook until the sugar is dissolved.

4. Adjust the seasonings, and serve over your favorite meat or soy loaf. Try it as a delicious topping for Stuffed Tofu (page 83).

TAKE A CHANCE:

• Use Chicken Broth (page 58) instead of vegetable.

One cook's sauce is another cook's gravy. Enhanced by the unique flavor of caraway seeds, this rich, wonderful blend of ingredients has a sweet-and-sour taste.

$2^1/4$ cups Vegetable Broth (page 59)

3 yellow or white onions, finely chopped

3 tablespoons arrowroot

1 teaspoon caraway seeds

2 teaspoons white vinegar

1 teaspoon date sugar

$1/4$ teaspoon freshly ground black pepper

Onion Gravy Croatia

Rich with onions, this gravy's secret ingredient is dry red wine. We like to serve this over Stuffed Burgers that have been made into mini loaves (page 92).

2$^1/_4$ cups Vegetable Broth (page 59)

1 large yellow or white onion, finely chopped

5 tablespoons unbleached flour

$^1/_2$ cup dry red wine

$^1/_4$ teaspoon freshly ground black pepper

YIELD: $^3/_4$ CUP   PREPARATION TIME: 30 MINUTES

1. Place $^1/_4$ cup of the broth in a skillet over medium heat. Add the onions and sauté 10 minutes, or until they begin to brown. Gradually add the flour, stirring constantly, until it is absorbed and begins to turn brown. Slowly add the remaining broth.

2. Bring the ingredients to a boil, then reduce the heat to medium-low. Add the wine and cook for 15 minutes, or until the gravy has thickened to the desired consistency.

TAKE A CHANCE:

• Use any combination of onions, shallots, and leeks.

• Use 3 tablespoons of arrowroot instead of the flour.

Chive Sauce Sweden

This sauce is a wonderful addition to just about any fish dish.

$^1/_4$ cup egg substitute

2 tablespoons fresh lemon juice

$^1/_2$ cup soy margarine, melted

3 tablespoons finely chopped chives

YIELD: $^3/_4$ CUP   PREPARATION TIME: 10 MINUTES

1. Whisk together egg substitute and lemon juice in a small bowl. Slowly add margarine while constantly whisking. Stir in chives.

2. Transfer the mixture to a small saucepan over medium-low heat. Stir constantly for 3 minutes, or just until the sauce begins to thicken.

3. Spoon the warm sauce over broiled fish or steamed vegetables.

TAKE A CHANCE:

• Use garlic chives instead of regular chives.

• Add $^1/_4$ teaspoon paprika or cayenne pepper to the sauce.

• Use 1 egg plus 2 egg whites in place of the egg substitute.

Scallion Sauce China

YIELD: 1 CUP   PREPARATION TIME: 1 HOUR

1. To make the scallion oil, place the safflower oil in a small skillet or wok over medium heat. Add the scallions and sauté until they begin to turn brown. Remove the scallions.

2. Add the soy sauce, water, and sugar, and bring to a boil while stirring constantly. Remove from the heat and let the sauce cool to room temperature.

3. Use the sauce immediately, or place it in a sealed container and refrigerate up to one week.

TAKE A CHANCE:

• Use 4 shallots or 1/4 cup any type of chopped onions instead of scallions.

• Use peanut oil to make the scallion oil.

The Chinese use very few sauces. We like the sweet, clean taste of this one that is the perfect dipping sauce for Scallion Bread (page 182). The scallion oil prepared in this recipe can substituted for the oil in most recipes.

1/2 cup shoyu or tamari soy sauce

3 tablespoons water

3 tablespoons date sugar

Scallion Oil

4 scallions, trimmed and cut into 2-inch pieces

1 cup safflower or light sesame oil

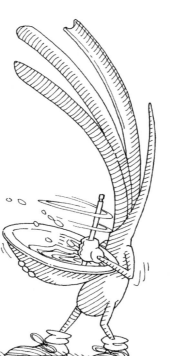

Berbere Sauce Ethiopia

*O*nions and garlic round out the flavor of this extra-spicy sauce used in Ethiopian cooking. It has hundreds of variations.

15 small dried red chili peppers

1 yellow or white onion, coarsely chopped

4 cloves garlic, coarsely chopped

1 cup water

Spice Blend

10 whole black peppercorns

2 tablespoons cayenne pepper

1 tablespoon paprika

2 teaspoons ground cumin

1 teaspoon ground cardamom

$^1/_2$ teaspoon ground ginger

$^1/_4$ teaspoon ground nutmeg

$^1/_4$ teaspoon ground cloves

YIELD: $1^1/_2$ CUPS   PREPARATION TIME: 25 MINUTES

1. Place the chili peppers in a heatproof bowl and cover with boiling water. Let stand about 20 minutes to soften. Remove and drain.

2. Place all of the spice blend ingredients in a hot, dry skillet and toast them for 2 minutes. Remove the pan from the heat.

3. Place the onions and garlic in a food processor and pulse 3 times. Add $^1/_4$ cup of the water and blend to form a paste. Add another $^1/_4$ cup of water and continue blending until smooth. Add the chilis, spices, and the remaining water, and continue to blend the ingredients to a thick purée.

4. Use immediately, or place in a sealed container and refrigerate up to 3 weeks.

TAKE A CHANCE:

• Omit the ground cardamom and use the seeds from 4 cardamom pods.

Trivial Tidbit

As far as we know, no one eating or wearing garlic has *ever* been bitten by a vampire.

Harissa Sauce Morocco

YIELD: ½ CUP   PREPARATION TIME: 1 HOUR

1. Place the chili peppers in a mixing bowl and cover with hot water. Cover the bowl and soak the chilies for 45 minutes to soften. Remove and drain.

2. Place the chilies, garlic, and lemon juice in a food processor and purée until smooth. Add additional lemon juice or oil for a thinner sauce.

3. Use the sauce immediately, or place it in a sealed container and refrigerate up to 10 days.

TAKE A CHANCE:

• Add 1 teaspoon curry powder.

• Add 10 pitted brine-cured black olives to the food processor

• For a sauce that is not quite as hot, remove the seeds from the chilies before soaking.

*S*erve this fiery sauce as a salad dressing, vegetable dip, or topping for crusty bread. We enjoy it alongside Couscous with Summer Vegetables (page 97).

½ cup small dried red chili peppers

5 cloves garlic, chopped

3 tablespoons fresh lemon juice

2 tablespoons extra-virgin olive oil

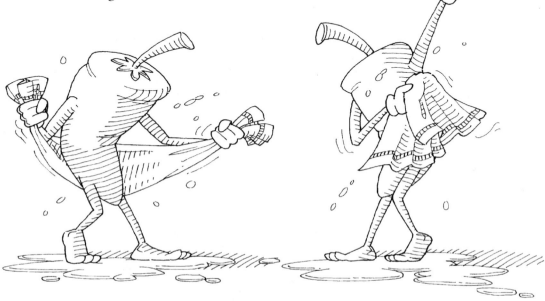

Garlic Chili Sauce Thailand

This sauce is pungent with garlic and hot chili peppers. Add some to a pot of soup or stew or to a marinade for chicken or fish.

5 cloves garlic

2 shallots, halved

6 red serrano or Thai chili peppers

1 tomato, seeded and chopped

2 tablespoons fresh lemon juice

YIELD: 1/2 CUP   PREPARATION TIME: 10 MINUTES

1. Place all of the ingredients in a food processor and blend until smooth. Add more lemon juice for a thinner sauce.

2. Use the sauce immediately, or place it in a sealed container and refrigerate up to 3 days.

TAKE A CHANCE:

• Use lime juice or fish sauce (available at Asian markets and gourmet shops) instead of lemon juice.

• Use roasted jalapeño chili peppers instead of Thai.

Skordalia Greece

In Greece, this garlic sauce is commonly served with boiled shrimp, baked fish, and steamed vegetables. Try it as a dip for raw vegetables.

2 baking potatoes, peeled and quartered

4 cloves garlic

1/2 cup extra-virgin olive oil

1/4 cup white vinegar

YIELD: 2 CUPS   PREPARATION TIME: 3 HOURS

1. Place the potatoes in a medium saucepan and cover with water. Bring to a boil and cook until fork tender. Drain.

2. Transfer the cooked potatoes to a food processor. Add the garlic and pulse 3 times. With the motor running, alternate adding the vinegar and oil in a slow stream. Blend into a smooth sauce. For a thinner sauce, add water in small amounts until the required consistency is achieved.

3. Spoon the sauce into a glass bowl or jar, cover, and refrigerate at least 2 hours before serving.

TAKE A CHANCE:

• Add 1 or 2 egg yolks for a richer sauce.

• Stir in 1/2 cup chopped almonds or walnuts before serving.

Creamy Roasted Garlic Sauce United States

YIELD: ³/₄ CUP   PREPARATION TIME: 15 MINUTES

1. Place the tofu in a food processor and pulse 3 times. Add the wine and garlic cloves, and pulse until smooth and creamy.
2. Transfer the sauce to a small saucepan. While stirring constantly, cook the sauce over low heat until it is thoroughly heated. If the sauce is too thick, add more wine.
3. Use the sauce immediately, or place it in a sealed container and refrigerate up to 2 days.

TAKE A CHANCE:

• Use Vegetable Broth (page 59) instead of wine.

We love the velvety texture of cream sauces but hate what it does to the waistline. So we came up with this luscious creamy garlic sauce using silken tofu. Rich, smooth taste without the high fat.

3 ounces silken tofu, drained

¹/₃ cup dry white wine

2 heads Roasted Garlic (page 25)

2 teaspoons soy margarine

Garlic Chili Paste Peru

YIELD: ¹/₂ CUP   PREPARATION TIME: 1 HOUR

1. Place the chili peppers in a heatproof bowl and cover with boiling water. Let stand about 45 minutes to soften the peppers thoroughly. Remove and drain.
2. Place the garlic and softened chili peppers in a food processor with ¹/₂ teaspoon of the olive oil, and process until smooth. Add the remaining oil and process for 1 minute.
3. Use the paste immediately, or place it in a sealed container and refrigerate up to 2 weeks.

TAKE A CHANCE:

• Freeze the paste in tablespoon-size portions for future use.

No less lethal than its Thai counterpart, this paste can be added to tofu, chicken, and fish dishes for a definite "pick-me-up." Covered and stored in the refrigerator, this paste will keep up to 2 weeks. Frozen, it will keep for months.

¹/₂ cup dried serrano or Thai chili peppers

6 cloves garlic

2 tablespoons extra-virgin olive oil

Garlic Spread Italy

This flavorful spread can turn an ordinary loaf of bread into a garlicky delight.

4 cloves garlic, crushed

1/2 cup soy margarine

YIELD: 1/2 CUP   PREPARATION TIME: 1 HOUR

1. Mix the garlic and margarine together in a small bowl until well-blended.
2. Refrigerate about 1 hour, or until firm.

TAKE A CHANCE:

• For extra zing, add a little paprika or cayenne pepper to the spread.

Garlic Mayonnaise France / Spain

Called aioli in France and ali-oli in Spain, this garlic-flavored mayonnaise is delicious on cooked vegetables and fish. Be sure to try it on Garlic Shrimp Appetizers (page 31).

4 cloves garlic, crushed

1 large egg

3 tablespoons fresh lemon juice

1 teaspoon dry mustard

1/8 teaspoon freshly ground black pepper

1/4 cup extra-virgin olive oil

YIELD: 1/2 CUP   PREPARATION TIME: 5 MINUTES

1. Place all of the ingredients, except the olive oil, in a food processor and blend until smooth. With the motor running, add the oil in a very slow stream and blend until creamy.
2. Use immediately, or transfer the mayonnaise to a glass jar. Cover and refrigerate up to 2 days.

TAKE A CHANCE:

• Stir the crushed garlic into 1/4 cup commercial nonfat mayonnaise. Allow the mixture to sit for 30 minutes before using.

• Experiment with different flavored oils for different tastes.

Shallot Spread France

YIELD: ½ CUP   PREPARATION TIME: 1 HOUR

1. Mix the shallots and margarine together in a small bowl until well-blended.

2. Refrigerate about 1 hour, or until firm.

TAKE A CHANCE:

• For chive spread, use 2 teaspoons chopped chives instead of garlic. For scallion spread, use 2 teaspoons chopped scallions.

A simple dab of this spread adds delicate flavor to cooked vegetables. Tightly covered and refrigerated, it will stay for several days.

2 large shallots, finely chopped

½ cup soy margarine

Rouille France

YIELD: ¾ CUP   PREPARATION TIME: 10 MINUTES

1. Remove the crusts and cut the bread into ½-inch slices. Place the slices in a strainer and moisten with cold water. When the bread is soaked through, squeeze out the water and set aside.

2. Place the garlic and chili pepper in a food processor and purée. Add the bread and pulse 3 times to blend. With the motor running, slowly add the oil and blend until the thick mixture is fairly creamy. Add the black pepper and pulse 3 times to mix.

3. Use immediately or transfer the sauce to a glass jar. Cover and refrigerate up to 3 days.

TAKE A CHANCE:

• Use 3 tablespoons chopped onion instead of garlic.

Sometimes described as hot mayonnaise, this fiery sauce is made with bread rather than eggs. Try a spoonful with your favorite vegetables or broiled fish, and be sure to add some to our Garlic Broth (page 60).

2 slices firm bread, such as sourdough or French

4 cloves garlic

1 fresh serrano or Thai chili pepper, seeded

¼ cup extra-virgin olive oil

¼ teaspoon freshly ground black pepper

Pesto Sauce Italy

*P*ungent *with garlic, this flavorful sauce goes well on any pasta salad or entrée. Lemon juice gives it a light taste. Try a dollop on Vegetable Kebabs (page 148) or Roasted Vidalias (page 135).*

4 cloves garlic

$^1/_2$ cup pine nuts

3 cups fresh basil leaves

$^1/_2$ cup fresh lemon juice

$^1/_2$ cup extra-virgin olive oil

$^1/_4$ cup freshly grated
   Parmesan cheese

YIELD: 3 CUPS   PREPARATION TIME: 10 MINUTES

1. Place the garlic and pine nuts in a food processor, and pulse until both are finely chopped. Add the basil and continue to pulse.

2. Add the lemon juice and continue to pulse until the ingredients are well-mixed. With the motor running, add the oil in a slow stream. Add the cheese and pulse until blended.

3. Use the pesto immediately, or place it in a sealed container and refrigerate it up to 2 days. You can freeze the pesto even longer.

TAKE A CHANCE:

• Use parsley or cilantro instead of basil.

• Use walnuts or almonds instead of pine nuts.

• To make Cream Cheese Pesto Spread, mix $^1/_2$ cup Pesto Sauce with 6 ounces softened nonfat cream cheese. Serve on crackers.

Gremolata Middle East

*I*f you're looking for something *to spice up a dish, this is it. Gremolata is a refreshing and colorful garnish for almost any dish.*

3 cloves garlic, finely chopped

2 tablespoons finely chopped
   lemon zest

2 tablespoons finely chopped
   fresh parsley

YIELD: $^1/_4$ CUP   PREPARATION TIME: 5 MINUTES

1. Using a fork, toss all of the ingredients together in a small bowl.

2. Use to garnish any dish that needs a little zip.

3. Store in the refrigerator for up to a week.

TAKE A CHANCE:

• Add 1 teaspoon of chopped walnuts or crushed red pepper to the mixture.

Hot Garlic Vinegar American Southwest

YIELD: 1 QUART   PREPARATION TIME: 3 WEEKS

1. Place the garlic and chili peppers in a sterilized quart jar with a tight-fitting lid. Add the vinegar, cover, and store in a cool, dark place for 3 weeks.

2. Strain the vinegar before using. Store any unused portion in the pantry or refrigerator. You can also add some chili peppers to the flavored vinegar for decoration.

TAKE A CHANCE:

• Add sprigs of fresh herbs, such as tarragon, rosemary, and oregano, to the vinegar for added flavor.

• Use cider vinegar instead of white vinegar.

Like oil, vinegar can be distinctively flavored with garlic. Use this vinegar as a base for salad dressings and marinades.

8 cloves garlic

1/2 cup serrano or Thai chili peppers

3 cups distilled white vinegar

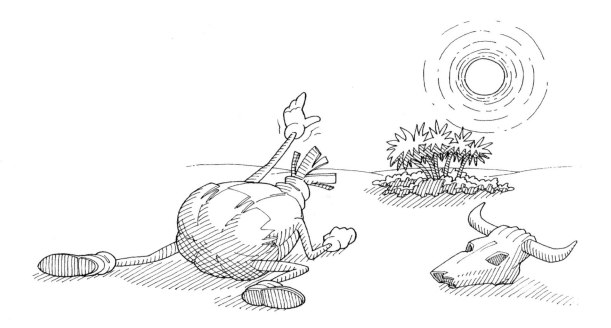

Garlic-Infused Olive Oil France / Italy

Use as a dipping sauce for Bruschetta (page 188) or serve as a warm sauce over pasta. We use extra-virgin olive oil, but feel free to use your favorite oil. (Note: Unless prepared and stored properly, garlic-infused oil can cause botulism. Be sure to read About Garlic-Infused Oils below.)

1/2 cup extra-virgin olive oil

12 cloves garlic, coarsely chopped

YIELD: 1/2 CUP   PREPARATION TIME: 1 HOUR

1. Place the olive oil in a small saucepan over low heat. Add the garlic and cook for 5 minutes. Remove the pan from the heat and allow the oil to come to room temperature.

2. Use the oil immediately, or place it in a sealed container and refrigerate up to 10 days. (If you remove the garlic, the oil will keep up to one month in the refrigerator.)

TAKE A CHANCE:

• Add a sprig of your favorite fresh herb, such as rosemary, thyme, or oregano, to the garlic as it cooks.

• To make Roasted Garlic-Infused Olive Oil, use 2 heads of roasted garlic instead of raw.

ABOUT GARLIC-INFUSED OILS

Bottles of garlic-infused oil make great gifts for all of the cooks on your gift-giving list. But unless you know that the oil will be stored in the refrigerator or used within a week or so, the garlic must be acidified before it is added to the oil. Infused oils that are improperly stored can cause botulism. Commercial garlic-in-oil products have been prohibited by the United States Food and Drug Administration unless the garlic has been acidified to levels below pH 4.6.

To acidify garlic at home, place whole, peeled cloves in full-strength vinegar and let them sit for 24 hours at room temperature. Remove the garlic and dry on paper toweling. Place the cloves in sterile jars and cover with your favorite oil—canola, corn, olive, safflower, and soybean are good choices. Seal the jar tightly. This oil can now be refrigerated or stored at room temperature.

Onion & Garlic Chutney India

1. Mix all of the ingredients, except the lemon juice, together in a medium bowl. Add the lemon juice and mix well.

2. Use immediately, or place in a sealed container and refrigerate up to 2 days.

TAKE A CHANCE:

• Place all of the ingredients in a food processor and pulse 3 or 4 times until just blended. Or continue to blend until a purée is formed.

• Use paprika instead of cayenne pepper.

• Cool the heat by adding ¹/₄ cup coarsely chopped cucumber.

Served as an accompaniment to curry dishes, this hot condiment should be used in very small amounts. Try it with Baked Rice (page 99) or Vindaloo (page 112).

1 yellow or white onion, coarsely chopped

12 cloves garlic, finely chopped

4 fresh jalapeño or serrano chili peppers, finely chopped

1 cup finely chopped fresh cilantro

¹/₂ teaspoon cayenne pepper

3 tablespoons fresh lemon juice

Scallion Paint Brushes France

These simple accompaniments add a decorative touch to any meal. You can also serve them alone as appetizers.

8 scallions, ends trimmed

Cold water

YIELD: 8 BRUSHES   PREPARATION TIME: 45 MINUTES

1. With a sharp knife, make $1/4$-inch-deep criss-cross cuts in the base of each scallion. Run your finger across the cuts to separate them.

2. Place the scallions in a large flat pan or container and cover with cold water. Cover and refrigerate for 30 minutes.

3. Remove the scallions and pat them dry with paper toweling. Again, run your fingers across the cuts to separate them. (The ends should be curled slightly, giving the scallions a "brush" look.)

4. Serve immediately or cover and store in the refrigerator overnight.

TAKE A CHANCE:

• Make leek paint brushes in the same manner, only make the criss-cross cuts about $1/2$-inch deep. Just be sure to wash the leeks thoroughly to remove the grit and sand.

Braised Chive Bundles United States

YIELD: 2 BUNDLES PREPARATION TIME: 15 MINUTES

1. Melt the margarine in a small skillet over medium heat. Add the pepper slices and sauté them for 5 minutes or until they are very soft. With a slotted spoon, transfer the peppers to a plate.

2. Place the chives in the skillet, making sure they are all facing the same direction. Carefully sauté them for 1 minute, rolling the entire bunch in the same direction at once. Remove the skillet form the heat.

3. Using a pair of tongs, remove half of the chives to the serving platter. Place one of the pepper strips across the middle of the chives and tuck the ends under the bundle. Repeat with the remaining chives and pepper strip.

TAKE A CHANCE:

• Used scallions instead of chives.

• Use slices of roasted red peppers instead of sautéed.

These delicate bundles of joy serve as colorful garnish on finished platters. Use them to brighten up Chicken with 40 Cloves of Garlic (page 114) or Baked Fish with Onions & Tomato Sauce (page 115).

1 tablespoon soy margarine

2 slices red bell pepper, $1/4$-inch thick and 2 inches long

1 large bunch chives, at least 3 inches long

Chapter 9

Mouthwatering Breads

Bread that is baking in the oven always fills the air with warm aromas to soothe the heart. Adding a little onion or garlic to the dough, soothes the soul as well. Like the Pied Piper, when baking these breads, you'll find anyone who is downwind attracted to the kitchen, where they'll gather to eagerly consume these savory loaves while they are still warm from the oven.

Onion Rounds Israel

Chopped onions crown the top of this stunning bread.

1 tablespoon active dry yeast

1 cup warm water

2 teaspoons date sugar

3$^{1}/_{2}$ cups unbleached white flour

2 teaspoons soy margarine, melted

1 cup coarsely chopped yellow or white onion

$^{1}/_{2}$ teaspoon paprika

YIELD: TWO 9-INCH ROUNDS   PREPARATION TIME: 2 HOURS

1. In a large mixing bowl, dissolve the yeast and sugar in $^{1}/_{2}$ cup of the water. Let stand for 10 minutes.

2. Add the remaining water and 2 cups of the flour and beat until smooth. Add the remaining flour, $^{1}/_{2}$ cup at a time, mixing until a soft dough forms. Turn the dough onto a lightly floured work surface and knead until smooth and elastic.

3. Form the dough into a ball and place it in a large bowl that is coated with oil or a nonstick spray. Turn the dough over to coat both sides. Cover the bowl with wax paper and a clean towel, and set it in a warm place for 1 hour, or until the dough doubles in size.

4. When the dough has doubled in size, punch it down and divide it in half.

5. Lightly coat two 9-inch-round cake pans with cooking spray. Press a piece of dough into each pan and coat the tops with melted margarine. Press the onions into the top of the dough and sprinkle with paprika.

6. Bake in a 450°F oven for 25 minutes, or until browned.

7. Serve warm.

TAKE A CHANCE:

• Garnish the loaves with 2 teaspoons caraway seeds before baking.

• Use whole wheat flour instead of unbleached white.

Onion Flat Bread Russia

YIELD: 12 FLAT BREADS   PREPARATION TIME: 30 MINUTES

1. Place 2 tablespoons of the water in a large bowl. Sprinkle the yeast over the water, then stir well. Let stand for 10 minutes, or until the mixture turns foamy.

2. Melt the margarine in a medium skillet over low heat. Add the onions and sauté for 5 minutes, or until soft. Remove the pan from the heat and let cool.

3. Stir the onions, the remaining water, and $^1/_2$ cup of the flour into the yeast mixture and beat until smooth. Add the remaining flour, $^1/_2$ cup at a time, mixing until a soft dough forms. Turn the dough onto a lightly floured work surface and knead until smooth and elastic.

4. Divide the dough into 12 equal pieces. With a floured rolling pin, flatten each piece of dough into a 6- to 8-inch circle.

5. Place a 10-inch skillet over medium–high heat and heat up until a drop of water sizzles and evaporates when sprinkled on the surface. Place a circle of dough in the pan and cook 12 to 15 seconds, or until the dough is browned on the bottom. Turn over and brown the other side. (It is very easy to burn this bread. If it starts to smoke, reduce the heat to medium and cook the dough a few seconds longer.)

6. Remove the bread from the pan and place on a wire rack to cool. Repeat with the remaining circles.

7. Serve immediately.

TAKE A CHANCE:

- Use chopped scallions instead of onions.

- Sauté 2 seeded, chopped jalapeño peppers along with the onions.

In a hurry? This onion-studded bread is actually made in a skillet on top of the stove.

$^1/_2$ cup warm water

1 package fast-rising active dry yeast

2 tablespoons soy margarine

1$^1/_2$ cups coarsely chopped yellow or white onions

2 cups unbleached white flour

Scallion Bread China

Also called scallion pancakes, buns, or coils, this flat bread is cooked on the stove. We find it perfect to serve with Bean Curd Kung Pao (page 90).

1 1/2 cups unbleached white
   flour

1/2 cup hot water

2 cups chopped scallions

1/2 teaspoon canola oil

1/4 cup peanut oil

YIELD: 8 BREADS   PREPARATION TIME: 45 MINUTES

1. Place the flour in a large mixing bowl, add the water, and mix until the dough forms a ball. Add a little more water if the dough is too stiff.

2. Turn the dough onto a lightly floured work surface and knead until very smooth.

3. Divide the dough into 8 equal pieces. With a floured rolling pin, flatten each piece of dough into an 8-x-2-inch rectangle. using a brush or the back of a spoon, lightly coat each strip with a little canola oil, then sprinkle with some scallions. Roll up the strips lengthwise, and pinch the ends together. Coil each strip to form a round. With the rolling pin or the palm of your hand, flatten each round to a 4-inch diameter.

4. Place the peanut oil in a large skillet over medium-high heat. Place as many pancakes in the pan as will fit in a single layer. Cook 2 to 3 minutes on each side, or until golden brown.

5. Remove the cooked pancakes and place on paper toweling to absorb any excess oil. Serve immediately as an appetizer or an accompaniment to a main dish.

TAKE A CHANCE:

• Roll the dough into one large rectangle. Top with the scallions and roll up. Coil the roll to form one large pancake. Cook as instructed above, adjusting the cooking time as necessary.

• Sprinkle the pancake with sesame seeds before cooking.

• Serve with Scallion Sauce (page 165) on the side.

Onion & Garlic Muffins Cuba

1. In a small bowl, mix together the onion, garlic, egg, milk, and margarine. Set aside.

2. In a large bowl, combine the flour, baking powder, and Sucanat. Add the onion mixture and stir only until the ingredients are mixed. Do not overstir. The batter should still have a few lumps.

3. Lightly coat a muffin tin with nonstick spray. Spoon the batter into the muffin tin, filling each cup two-thirds full.

4. Bake in a 400°F oven for 15 to 20 minutes, or until a toothpick inserted in the center of a muffin comes out clean. Remove the muffins from the tin, place them on a wire rack, and cool 5 minutes before serving.

TAKE A CHANCE:

• Make the muffins using all onion or all garlic.

• Substitute all or part of the onion and garlic with shallots and leeks.

• Sprinkle the batter-filled muffin cups with 2 teaspoons finely chopped chives before baking.

These moist, rich-tasting muffins are perfect accompaniments for Hot Island Chicken (page 110) or Broiled Tuna with Garlic & Shallot Marinade (page 120).

1 yellow or white onion, finely chopped

3 cloves garlic, finely chopped

1/4 cup egg substitute

1 cup skim milk

1/4 cup melted soy margarine

2 cups unbleached white flour

3 teaspoons baking powder

1 1/2 teaspoons Sucanat or 1 teaspoon date sugar

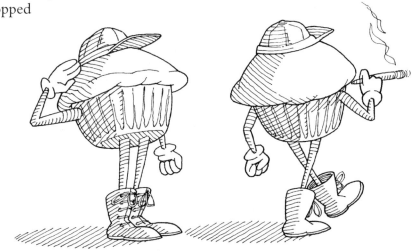

Chive Biscuits United States

Thoughts of summer gardens abound when eating these luscious chive-flecked morsels. Top them with some Red Onion Spread (page 16) or serve them alongside Wrapped Tofu (page 82).

2 cups unbleached white flour

1 tablespoon baking powder

3 tablespoons finely chopped fresh chives

1/4 cup canola oil

3/4 cup skim milk

YIELD: 15 BISCUITS   PREPARATION TIME: 30 MINUTES

1. Mix together the flour, baking powder, and chives in a large bowl. Add the oil and mix until the flour resembles coarse crumbs. Add the milk and mix to form a soft dough.

2. Turn the dough onto a lightly floured work surface and knead 5 or 6 times. Using a floured rolling pin, roll out the dough to a 1/2- to 3/4-inch thickness. Flour a 2-inch round cookie cutter, biscuit cutter, or the rim of a glass, and cut the dough into rounds. Gather the unused dough, roll it out, and cut more rounds.

3. Place the rounds on an ungreased cookie sheet, and place in a 450°F oven for 10 minutes, or until the biscuits begin to brown.

4. Remove from the oven and serve hot.

TAKE A CHANCE:

- Use 1 cup unbleached white flour and 1 cup whole wheat flour.

- Use 2 tablespoons chopped chive blossoms instead of stems.

Onion Cheese Cornbread American Southwest

YIELD: 9-INCH SQUARE CORNBREAD
PREPARATION TIME: 45 MINUTES

1. Mix together the cornmeal, flour, baking powder, and sugar in a large bowl. Stir in the eggs, milk, oil, and water and mix well. Add the onion, corn, and cheese.

2. Pour the batter into a 9-inch square baking pan that has been lightly coated with cooking spray. Using a spatula or the back of a spoon, spread the batter evenly.

3. Bake in a 425°F oven for 30 minutes, or until a toothpick inserted in the center of the bread comes out clean.

TAKE A CHANCE:

• Add 5 cloves crushed garlic.

• Add 4 chopped and seeded jalapeño chili peppers. The heat of these peppers will mellow somewhat with baking.

Filled with grated onions, rich cheese, and creamy corn, this bread is almost a meal in itself. Try it with Black Bean Salad (page 49).

2 1/2 cups yellow cornmeal

1 cup unbleached white flour

3 teaspoons baking powder

3 teaspoons date sugar

3 eggs, lightly beaten

1/2 cup skim milk

1/2 cup safflower oil

1 cup water

3/4 cup grated yellow or white onion

2 cups cream-style corn

1 3/4 cups grated sharp cheddar cheese

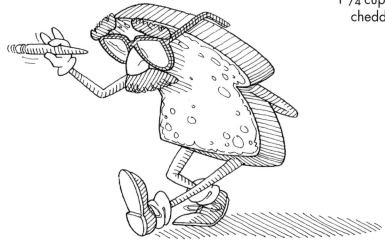

Onion Focaccia Italy

Topped with slow-cooked onions and shallots, this satisfying bread goes well with any meal. Because it can be served at room temperature, it is a great take-along bread for a party or picnic.

Dough

1 package active dry yeast

1 cup warm water

2 tablespoons extra-virgin olive oil

1½ cups whole wheat pastry flour

1¼ cups unbleached white flour

Topping

2 tablespoons soy margarine

2 yellow or white onions, thinly sliced

3 shallots, thinly sliced

1 teaspoon date sugar

YIELD: 12-INCH FLAT LOAF   PREPARATION TIME: 3 HOURS

1. To prepare the dough, place the yeast and water in a large mixing bowl and stir until the yeast is dissolved. Let stand for 10 minutes or until the mixture turns foamy.

2. Stir in the olive oil, then add the whole wheat flour ½ cup at a time, mixing well after each addition. Stir in the white flour ½ cup at a time, mixing until a soft dough forms.

3. Turn the dough onto a lightly floured work surface and knead for 10 minutes, or until the dough is smooth and elastic.

4. Form the dough into a ball and place it in a large bowl that is coated with oil or nonstick cooking spray. Turn the dough over to coat both sides. Cover the bowl with wax paper and a clean towel, and set it in a warm place for 45 minutes, or until the dough doubles in size.

5. While the dough is rising, make the topping. Melt the margarine in a large skillet over medium heat. Add the onions, shallots, and sugar, and sauté for 15 minutes, or until the onions begin to turn brown and caramelize. Remove from the heat and set aside.

6. When the dough has doubled in size, punch it down and knead for 2 minutes.

7. Lightly coat a 12-inch-round pan with cooking spray. Press the dough into the pan. Using a fork, poke holes in the dough at 1-inch intervals. Spread the caramelized onions on top. Cover the pan and let the dough rise for 45 minutes.

8. Bake in a 375°F oven for 20 minutes, or until the crust is golden brown. Serve at room temperature.

TAKE A CHANCE:

• Knead 2 tablespoons of minced fresh herbs into the dough.

• Top the focaccia with Mess O'Onions (page 126) before baking.

Pissaladiere France

1. To make the dough, mix the yeast, Sucanat, and $^1/_2$ cup of the water together in a large bowl. Set aside for 10 minutes, or until the mixture turns foamy.

2. Add the remaining water to the bowl, and stir in $^1/_2$ cup of flour at a time, mixing well until a soft dough forms. Turn the dough onto a lightly floured work surface and knead until smooth and elastic.

3. Form the dough into a ball and place it in a large bowl that is coated with oil or nonstick spray. Turn the dough over to coat both sides. Cover the bowl with wax paper and a clean towel, and set it in a warm place for 1 hour, or until the dough doubles in size.

4. While the dough is rising, make the topping. Place the broth and 1 tablespoon of the oil in a large skillet over medium heat. Add the onions and sauté for 15 minutes, or until the onions are soft and golden brown. Remove from the heat and set aside.

5. When the dough has doubled in size, punch it down and knead for 2 minutes.

6. Lightly coat a 12-inch tart pan with nonstick cooking spray. Press the dough into the pan. Spread the sautéed onions on top. Arrange the anchovies on top of the onions to form a lattice design. Place an olive in the center of each lattice square. Drizzle the remaining oil on top.

7. Bake in a 400°F oven for 20 minutes, or until the crust is golden brown.

8. Serve hot or warm.

TAKE A CHANCE:

• Add 6 finely chopped garlic cloves to the topping.

• Serve the topping on your favorite pizza crust or pie dough.

Slow-cooked onions, flavorful anchovies, and black Niçoise olives are the starring ingredients in this wonderful bread from Provence. Serve it with Poached Chicken Salad Aioli (page 56) or Vegetable Soup Pistou (page 69).

Dough

1 package dry yeast

1 teaspoon Sucanat or 1 teaspoon date sugar

1 cup warm water

$3^1/_2$ cups unbleached white flour

Topping

3 tablespoons Vegetable Broth (page 59)

3 tablespoons extra-virgin olive oil

4 yellow or white onions, thinly sliced

12 flat anchovy fillets, cut into thin strips

$^1/_2$ cup pitted black Niçoise olives

Classic Garlic Bread Italy

Crusty Italian bread topped with a spread of garlic and herbs is an elegant accompaniment to any meal.

1 loaf Italian bread

1 recipe Garlic Spread (page 170)

1/2 teaspoon dried oregano

1/4 teaspoon paprika

2 teaspoons freshly grated Parmesan cheese

YIELD: 8 SLICES   PREPARATION TIME: 15 MINUTES

1. Cut the bread in half lengthwise and evenly coat each half with Garlic Spread. Place on a baking sheet. Sprinkle the remaining ingredients on top.

2. Bake in a 350°F oven for 10 minutes, or until the butter begins to melt and the bread becomes crisp. Serve hot.

TAKE A CHANCE:

• Instead of cutting the loaf in half, cut it into individual 1-inch-thick slices. Add the spread and toppings, then assemble the slices back into a loaf shape before baking.

• Top the bread with thin slices of mozzarella cheese.

• Use pita or sourdough bread instead of Italian.

Bruschetta Italy

This bread's great taste comes from rubbing whole cloves of garlic over its surface. Serve plain or topped with Eggplant Caponata (page 53).

8 slices Italian bread, 1/2-inch thick

8 cloves garlic

1/4 cup Garlic-Infused Olive Oil (page 174)

YIELD: 8 SLICES   PREPARATION TIME: 15 MINUTES

1. Toast the bread on both sides. Rub each toasted slice with a garlic clove until the clove disappears.

2. Serve the bread with Garlic-Infused Olive Oil (page 174) to use as a dip.

TAKE A CHANCE:

• Toast the bread on the barbecue

• After rubbing in the garlic, rub a piece of tomato over each piece of bread.

Indian Fry Bread American Southwest

YIELD: 8 PIECES PREPARATION TIME: 30 MINUTES

1. Place the flour and baking powder in a large bowl. Add the water and mix until a soft dough forms. Turn the dough onto a lightly floured board and knead until it is smooth and elastic. If the dough is sticky, add more flour.

2. Shape the dough into balls about 2-inches in diameter. Roll out the balls until they are about $1/4$- to $1/2$-inch thick.

3. Place about 2 inches of oil in a skillet that is just large enough to hold a piece of the flattened dough. Heat the oil over medium-high heat then add a piece of the dough. Fry the bread on both sides until it is puffed and browned. Remove from the skillet and place on paper toweling. Fry the remaining pieces of dough.

4. Top with Mess O'Onions and serve immediately.

TAKE A CHANCE:

• Crown this bread with any of the sauces or toppings found in this book.

• Omit Mess O' Onions and serve with honey on the side.

Okay, your cholesterol count is fine, and you've saved your calorie count for this traditional fry bread topped with Mess O' Onions.

3 cups unbleached white flour

1 tablespoon baking powder

$1^1/3$ cups warm water

1 cup shortening or vegetable oil

2 cups Mess O'Onions (page 126)

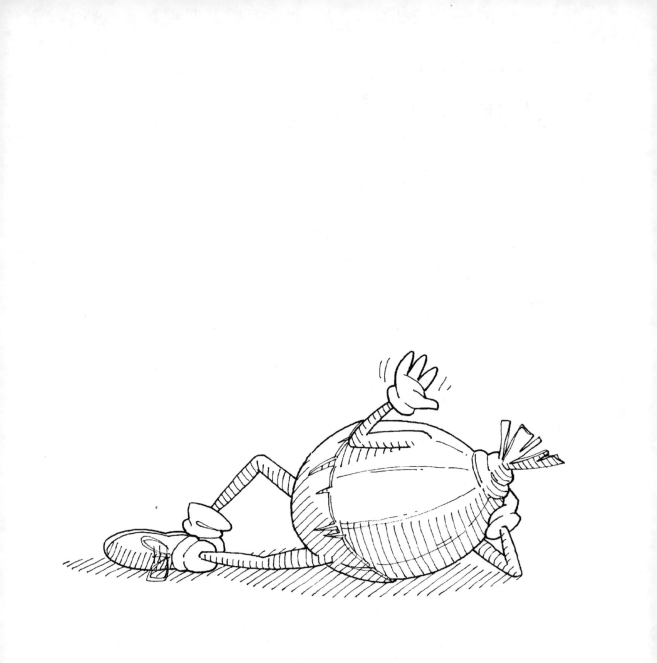

Index

Metric Conversion Tables

Common Liquid Conversions

Measurement	=	Milliliters
1/4 teaspoon	=	1.25 milliliters
1/2 teaspoon	=	2.50 milliliters
3/4 teaspoon	=	3.75 milliliters
1 teaspoon	=	5.00 milliliters
1 1/4 teaspoons	=	6.25 milliliters
1 1/2 teaspoons	=	7.50 milliliters
1 3/4 teaspoons	=	8.75 milliliters
2 teaspoons	=	10.0 milliliters
1 tablespoon	=	15.0 milliliters
2 tablespoons	=	30.0 milliliters

Measurement	=	Liters
1/4 cup	=	0.06 liters
1/2 cup	=	0.12 liters
3/4 cup	=	0.18 liters
1 cup	=	0.24 liters
1 1/4 cups	=	0.30 liters
1 1/2 cups	=	0.36 liters
2 cups	=	0.48 liters
2 1/2 cups	=	0.60 liters
3 cups	=	0.72 liters
3 1/2 cups	=	0.84 liters
4 cups	=	0.96 liters
4 1/2 cups	=	1.08 liters
5 cups	=	1.20 liters
5 1/2 cups	=	1.32 liters

Converting Fahrenheit to Celsius

Fahrenheit	=	Celsius
200—205	=	95
220—225	=	105
245—250	=	120
275	=	135
300—305	=	150
325—330	=	165
345—350	=	175
370—375	=	190
400—405	=	205
425—430	=	220
445—450	=	230
470—475	=	245
500	=	260

Conversion Formulas

LIQUID When You Know	Multiply By	To Determine
teaspoons	5.0	milliliters
tablespoons	15.0	milliliters
fluid ounces	30.0	milliliters
cups	0.24	liters
pints	0.47	liters
quarts	0.95	liters

WEIGHT When You Know	Multiply By	To Determine
ounces	28.0	grams
pounds	0.45	kilograms